Let sleeping dogs lie?

What men should know before getting tested for prostate cancer

Simon Chapman, Alexandra Barratt and Martin Stockler

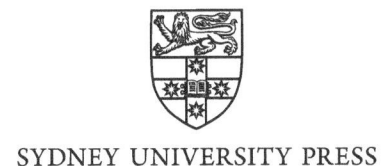

SYDNEY UNIVERSITY PRESS

Published 2010 by SYDNEY UNIVERSITY PRESS
University of Sydney Library
sydney.edu.au/sup

National Library of Australia Cataloguing-in-Publication entry

Author: Chapman, Simon, 1951-
Title: Let sleeping dogs lie? : what men should know before getting tested for
            prostate cancer / Simon Chapman, Alexandra Barratt and Martin Stockler.
ISBN: 9781920899684 (pbk.)
Notes: Includes bibliographical references and index.
Subjects: Prostate--Cancer--Australia--Treatment--Complications.
            Prostate--Diseases--Treatment--Complications.
            Men--Medical examinations--Australia.
            Medical screening--Australia.
            Men--Health and hygiene.
Other Authors/Contributors:
            Barratt, Alexandra, 1960-
            Stockler, Martin.
Dewey Number: 616.65

Cover design by Miguel Yamin, the University Publishing Service

Contents

Why have we written this book?

We will all die one day. Death itself cannot be prevented, though the time at which we die may be postponed through effective prevention and treatment. But many people invest huge emotional energy in the idea that their eventual cause of death might somehow be avoided. The very Australian idea of the "good innings" often gets lost in all this. If you ask people to imagine their preferred form of death, many talk about something "quick" where there would be no time to anticipate what lay ahead and no pain. However, most would talk about peacefully dying in their sleep, at a late stage in life, after a life largely free of disease and disability, allowing them to enjoy their later years with good mobility, free of pain, having seen their family and grandchildren grow up, and leaving their affairs in order. Such a death would probably mean dying suddenly from a heart attack or cerebrovascular disease (stroke).

Few people would ever nominate cancer as their preferred cause of death. Cancer and its recurrence [1] has become more feared than almost any other disease. Literature and cinema [2] are full of fearful references to cancer as a wasting, painful and ugly disease that slowly erodes the body, spreading inexorably and depressing everyone around the person suffering the disease. The word "cancer" has become a metaphor for something loathed, rotten and uncontrollable. We speak of cancer "invading" the body. We speak of a prevalent negative attitude or development as a "cancer" in the community. Crumbling buildings are said to have concrete cancer.

In 1971 US President Richard Nixon famously declared "war" on cancer [3], and the language of both cancer control and cancer patienthood is full of battle, heroic and stoic metaphors about struggles, fighting and defeating the disease [4, 5]. Cancer seems to attract such language more than any other disease and this has an impact on both the anticipated and lived experience of cancer.

Being told that you have cancer can be devastating: dreaded news that can preoccupy those diagnosed, seriously eroding quality of life, and causing depression [6]. Many cancer control agencies now refer to the experience of living with cancer as "the cancer journey". This journey always starts with the patient being told that they have cancer. Once that news has been received, it stays with you for the rest of your life. Being told that you have cancer is not trivial information. It holds potential to start a sometimes rapidly unfolding train of events that may fundamentally alter the course and quality of your life. The main goal is often to fight and defeat the cancer that has suddenly been announced as a very unwelcome intruder in your body. The cancer will typically be surgically attacked and/or bombarded with radiation and highly toxic chemotherapies, all in the cause of the self-evidently important goal of stopping it from killing you.

Against this, the idea that many men might have discoverable cancer in their bodies and yet may decide to not take steps to discover it is almost heretical to everything we have come to know about health, medicine and fighting disease. But this is a decision that many highly informed men are taking today about prostate cancer. Far from being simply dismissed as scared or ignorant screening "refusniks" – men who just need more support or persuasion to get tested – many men have taken what is for them a rational, evidence-based decision to choose to remain ignorant of whether they might already harbour prostate cancer in their bodies.

In taking this decision, these men are not eccentric mavericks but are in fact reflecting the overwhelming body of expert global consensus about whether it is a sensible thing to have all middle-aged and older men – apparently free of the disease (that is, with no symptoms) – routinely tested for prostate cancer. There are now a large number of expert cancer and other public health agencies which have assessed the net risks and benefits of screening large numbers of asymptomatic men for prostate cancer to see whether population-wide activity driven by such a policy would actually save lives.

Many governments have formally adopted policies of cancer screening in particular age groups for different diseases. In Australia, the Commonwealth government has formally adopted a policy of targeting screening for breast cancer in women aged 50–69 and colorectal cancer in people aged over 50. It has long advocated that sexually active women be screened for cervical cancer by having Pap smears.

While some prominent Australian urologists are very active in talking up the importance of prostate cancer screening, few Australians would be aware that no government anywhere in the world has a formal policy supporting prostate cancer screening. Nor would they be aware that aside from some professional urological societies, no reputable cancer control or expert prevention agency anywhere in the world currently recommends screening for the disease. Here are just a few illustrative examples:

- The Australian government's Australian Health Technology Advisory Committee examined the case for population screening for prostate cancer and in its 1997 report [7], did not recommend it. Thirteen years on, it has not changed that recommendation.

- No state Cancer Council nor their national body, the Cancer Council Australia supports screening: "The Cancer Council supports expert reviews that current evidence does not support population screening of well men for prostate cancer." [8]
- The Royal Australian College of General Practitioners: "Routine screening for prostate cancer with digital rectal examination (DRE), Prostate Specific Antigen (PSA) or transabdominal ultrasound is not recommended." [9]
- The American Cancer Society:

    The American Cancer Society recommends that men make an informed decision with their doctor about whether to be tested for prostate cancer. Research has not yet proven that the potential benefits of testing outweigh the harms of testing and treatment. The American Cancer Society believes that men should not be tested without learning about what we know and don't know about the risks and possible benefits of testing and treatment. [10]

- British Columbia's Cancer Agency in Canada:

    PSA testing is of unknown value as a population screening test. Although there is good evidence that it increases the detection rate of early stage, clinically significant prostate cancers, there is little evidence to date that such early detection leads to reduced mortality; the "gold standard" for evaluating screening tests. [11]

- The UK's National Screening Committee: "The UK NSC does not recommend screening men for prostate cancer." [12]
- The US Preventive Services Task Force:

    The USPSTF concludes that the current evidence is insufficient to assess the balance of benefits and harms of prostate cancer screening in men younger than age 75 years.

The USPSTF recommends against screening for prostate cancer in men age 75 years or older. [13]

- The Prostate Cancer Foundation of Australia (PFCA) is an example of one of the few agencies which do support screening. Its policy states:

  PCFA recommends that men at 50 with no family history of prostate cancer, and men at 40 with a family history, should seek voluntary annual assessments in the form of a Prostate Specific Antigen (PSA) blood test together with a Digital Rectal Examination (DRE). [14]

Despite this international expert consensus, *de facto* screening of populations is well under way, being driven by well-meaning advice about the importance of having men becoming more informed about their health. "Women have their cancer tests, men have theirs" runs the simplistic argument at its most basic level.

A 2003 review of the issue in the *Lancet* concluded that if one million men over 50 were screened,

> about 110,000 with raised PSAs will face anxiety of possible cancer, about 90,000 will undergo biopsy, and 20,000 will be diagnosed with cancer. If 10,000 of these men underwent surgery, about 10 would die of the operation, 300 will develop severe urinary incontinence and even in the best hands 4000 will become impotent.

And then came the crunch:

> The number of men whose prostate cancer would have impinged on their lives is unknown. [15]

This neat summary encapsulates why this issue is so important. Men are being increasingly urged by some to subject themselves to a medical procedure that may dramatically reduce their quality of life by causing impotence and incontinence. But the evidence that this procedure will in fact save men's lives is by no means well established, while the risks are known and very real.

By 2003 (the latest date from which published estimates are available), around 50% of Australian men aged 40 and over were estimated to have been tested for prostate cancer [16]. With high profile promotion of screening through campaigns like Movember, and men being urged to take the test by campaigns organised by the Prostate Cancer Foundation of Australia, this proportion would be considerably higher today in 2010. But many men consciously choose not to be tested.

This book tries to explain why many men make that decision. It seeks to bring their reasons out into the open, and repudiates the facile idea that men who elect not to be tested are nothing more than unmanly "pussies" who are squeamish about having a doctor put a finger up their rectum to feel for prostate enlargement or who are just indifferent to protecting their health. This sort of trivialising focus has been a prominent part of campaigns in Australia with slogans like "Be a man!" designed to get men to be screened. Comic actor Magda Szubanski, whose father died of the disease, told the national *60 Minutes* TV audience in 2007: "Don't be a pussy. Go and get the check" [17].

Our aim in this book is to provide a detailed examination of the main questions that a man should be asking before deciding to get tested. Deciding to have a PSA test can quickly lead to a course of events that for some men may save their life. But as we will show, for many more a test will result in serious, unnecessary surgery and other interventions. In a large proportion of cases, this will cause enduring and often permanent, major after-effects in the form of sexual impotence, urinary incontinence and less commonly, faecal incontinence. The surgery will have been unnecessary because – strange as this idea may seem – the cancer would have never caused problems in many of these men's lives. This is an absolutely central point that is at the heart of this book.

The other core point we will make is that medical science is today unable to predict with any precision which early discovered prostate cancers will turn out to be those that kill, and particularly which will kill men in middle age. Many people have deep faith in medical science. They believe that diagnostic tests undertaken by doctors and pathologists can provide highly reliable information that can predict with great precision the likely progress of a disease like cancer. Often, this is true and often people have experienced this when a diagnostic test has led to an effective form of therapy that has cured a disease in them or other family members. So when a much-promoted test turns out to have major shortcomings in its ability to accurately point to a cancer that urgently needs attention, it is understandable that many would find this news hard to believe. But as we will see (p58), the frontline diagnostic tool in efforts to screen for prostate cancer – the PSA test – is a tool which has very poor ability to find problematic cancers. It finds many benign cancers which could have been left alone.

Prostate cancer is the second most common cause of cancer death in Australian men (after lung cancer). Like deaths from nearly all forms of cancer – but even more so in the case of prostate cancer – the large majority of men who die from the disease die late in life (see p31) close to when they would have in all probability have died from another cause anyway. For many, the idea that one might decide to not take every possible step to catch this cancer early is nothing less than bizarre. But in the zeal to wage war on cancer, we now know there are many avoidable casualties: people who get caught up in whirlwind of unnecessary medical intervention from which it is difficult to withdraw.

In Australia today, there are many thousands of men who have had their prostates removed and who, as a result, are permanently sexually impotent (meaning that they are unable to attain an erection sufficient for intercourse). Some of these men, and others who are not impotent, also have ongoing incontinence problems. These are not problems that you wear on your sleeve, or announce to the world. They are typically endured privately and rationalised by the very powerful idea that these problems were small prices to have to pay to remain alive. A small minority of these men may be right in thinking this: but for having found their cancer early, and having their prostate removed, they might well be dead. But as we will see, there is a great number of individuals who have been treated unnecessarily for the disease. It would not have killed them and they now live with the consequences of having that unnecessary treatment.

Some men who have had their prostates surgically removed become determined and committed advocates for prostate cancer screening. Many see them as powerfully convincing, living proof-of-the-pudding that early detection saves lives. After all, they have lived to tell the tale. But as we shall explore, for every such man whose life was saved as a result of early detection, there can be up to 47 more [18] who in all probability would not have died as a result of the cancer that was found. For many of these men, their sexual impotence, their incontinence and their enduring anxiety that the cancer may have spread in undetectable ways and may return in other parts of their body are legacies that could have been avoided.

Australia has seen febrile, often acrimonious debate on prostate cancer screening. In February 2003, an interview with Professor Alan Coates, then chief executive of the Cancer Council Australia and aged 59, was published in the *Australian Financial Review*. He stated that he had personally chosen to not have a PSA test, arguing

[t]he test may find things that didn't need to be found or it may find things when it is too late to fix them. The supposition is that there is a group in between where it finds something early enough to make a real difference, but there is no proof that such a window of opportunity exists. [19]

The article generated widespread, overwhelmingly negative responses from several Australian urologists and cancer survivors, including two federal politicians who were incendiary in their criticism, particularly from within the safety of parliamentary privilege [20]. An editorial called Coates "the apostate professor" whose actions will have "confused thousands of men" [21]. Coates protested that to be an apostate, one must have once believed [22].

This very public row would have been noticed by millions of Australians used to encountering cancer control officials (including Coates) enthusiastically promoting population screening for cervical, breast and colorectal cancer, and stressing the importance of early detection. Yet here was one of the nation's most senior cancer experts saying that he personally had taken the decision to not be tested. Why, many would have asked, should the case for the early detection of prostate cancer be any different than for other cancers?

The message about the importance of early detection for saving lives has been driven home over many years through public awareness campaigns for many diseases. The idea has taken on something of the status of a commonsense law, admitting no challenge. Unsurprisingly, a recent study found that over two-thirds of Victorian adults believed their chances of surviving prostate cancer would be very much improved by early detection [23]. US survey evidence shows 87% of adults believe that routine cancer screening is almost always a good idea and that finding cancer early can save lives (74% said most or all of the time). Moreover, 77% of men said that they would try to keep having a PSA test even if a doctor recommended that they stopped having or had less frequent testing [24].

There are also studies that show that when men are better informed about prostate cancer their interest in screening goes down. For example, an Australian study considered men who were visiting their GP who were sent balanced information about the pros and cons of PSA screening. Before receiving the information, about 50% of men were definitely interested in being screened, but afterwards, only 24% reported being definitely interested [25]. In an earlier US study, men scheduled for a routine visit to their doctor were randomly divided into some who were shown a video about the pros and cons of PSA screening and others who did not watch the video. Men who saw the video were less likely to want the test afterwards, (30% in the video group, compared to 67% in the control group), and fewer went ahead with the test at the next opportunity (12% in the video group compared to 23% in the control group) [26]. There are two other studies like these, with similar findings [27, 28] and one [29] which found information about the pros and cons of screening made no difference to the percentage of men who chose to be screened.

A senior cancer control figure like Alan Coates publicly declaring that he personally would not be tested would thus have appeared to many as heretical and counterintuitive. But Coates was no Robinson Crusoe: he was not alone in his decision. Just as many men elect to be tested for prostate cancer, an equally if not larger number of well-informed men are today electing not to be tested on the basis of the currently available scientific evidence. Many make similar decisions to not undertake genetic screening for a range of diseases which may provide unwelcome information of doubtful use.

We have written this book to provide the hundreds of thousands of Australian men facing the decision about whether to get tested for prostate cancer with important information that many of them would not have encountered before. Public discussion about prostate cancer screening in Australia today is overwhelmingly dominated by pro-screening voices, many of whom have obvious vested interests in promoting widespread testing and medical intervention (see p112). As we will show, while it is almost standard for all parties to this debate to emphasise the vital importance of men being informed about the pros and cons of prostate cancer screening, attention to the "cons" has been woefully neglected or avoided by many actively promoting screening.

Prostate screening advocates often include men diagnosed and treated for prostate cancer, urologists and some non-government advocacy groups, including those supported by the manufacturers of prostate cancer diagnostic tests and treatments. These advocates have sometimes been aggressive in attacking those who have expressed reservations about the wisdom of screening [30]. In 2001, the editors of the US-based *Western Journal of Medicine* were subjected to particularly vicious lobbying and character assassination following cautious remarks they made in *The San Francisco Chronicle* newspaper about prostate cancer screening. Efforts were made to have them dismissed from their roles, and they were said to be promoting "geriatricide": the killing of aged men [31].

In 2003, when one of us (SC) wrote to a Federal Member of Parliament, Jim Lloyd, questioning a letter he had written to *The Sydney Morning Herald* claiming that "there was now less than a 4 per cent chance of incontinence" following treatment for prostate cancer, Mr Lloyd replied that "many academics place far too much reliance on statistics and forget the human aspects. Whilst you continue to study your surveys, figures and databases I will continue to deal with real issues." He included (with permission) a letter from Dr Phillip Katelaris (who said Lloyd was welcome to forward his letter to the press). Katelaris described SC as "a man quite divorced from the anguish of prostate cancer, a non-feeling egocentric 'past president of the

Australian Consumers' Association." This will give readers a flavour of both the sometimes very personal nature of the debate and the disdain that some have for evidence across large numbers of men, seemingly preferring to base health policy on the apparent benefits that have occurred for individual men who are personally convinced that prostate screening saves lives.

High profile campaigns like Movember reflect none of this debate. Movember's website states

> We want everyone to know that men over the age of 50, and those over 40 with a family history, are at risk of prostate cancer and encourage them to be tested annually because it is highly curable if detected and treated early. [32]

We often hear urologists and prostate cancer advocacy groups via campaigns like Movember urging that men should be screened. Far less often, we hear others urging that men should not rush into it and think very carefully about both the benefits and risks. All agree that it is a decision that should be talked over with one's doctor. But with waiting room queues putting pressure on a doctor's time, such conversations about such major decisions can often be rather short and leave a lot of questions unexplored.

In this book we will examine what is actually meant by being "at risk" for prostate cancer and also the evidence driving the proposal that men should be tested every year for the disease. We will look in detail at the results of a nine-year multi-nation European trial published in 2009 [18] and a 14-year Swedish trial published in 2010 [33, 34] which sought to answer the question of whether men who are screened for prostate cancer have a lower death rate from the disease than men who do not get screened. We will look at very recent evidence from Australia about what men undergoing treatment for prostate cancer can expect in terms of continuing sexual function and continence. Finally, we will look at claims made by some surgeons about the alleged greatly reduced risks of impotence and incontinence when "robotic" surgical techniques are used in laparoscopic ("keyhole") surgery for prostate cancer. As we will see, men should treat these claims with a good deal of circumspection.

Finally, we feel it is important to say something about claims that are often made about "percentage change" in outcomes like death or adverse side effects. There are two ways that change can be expressed in ordinary language: relative change and absolute change. Consider the case of smoking. Imagine if in the first year of a study 25% of adults smoked, and 10 years later, when the same group were again questioned, 18% now smoked. The absolute difference between 25 and 18 is 7% or a fall of 1.43% per year. But the relative difference is 28% or 2.8% a year (a reduction of 7% off a baseline of 25% is 28% less). Twenty-eight per cent sounds more impressive and is likely to be the figure that anyone would select who wanted to "talk up" the improvement. Those wanting to talk down the progress to reduce smoking – for example, to argue for stronger legislation and campaign funding – would probably emphasise the absolute, smaller figure in an effort to promote concern that not enough was being done.

Those selecting absolute or relative measures are often not explicit in what they say, particularly when a complex study is reported in the news media in just a few sentences. We have often noticed this in public discussions about prostate cancer. Sydney man-about-town, lawyer and newspaper columnist Charles Waterstreet wrote in his Sunday newspaper column in November 2009 that "Extensive PSA screening in other countries has meant a 40 per cent fall in the mortality rate" [35]. Newspaper writers rarely cite their sources, and Waterstreet was no exception here. But if he was referring to the 2009 *New England Journal of Medicine* European trial [18], the claim for "40% fall in mortality" is quite misleading. The fall was 20% in relative terms derived from data obtained over nine years of follow-up that showed there were 2.94 deaths per 1000 men in the group of screened men compared with 3.65 deaths per 1000 men in nine years (see p98).

A recent US survey [36] of medical decisions specifically looked at the decision US men made with their doctors about PSA screening. The survey included 375 men who had been tested in the previous two years (85%) and men who had discussed having the test but had not actually gone ahead with the test (15%). Of these men, 70% reported their doctor had discussed the test with them before a decision about testing was made; 94% said the doctor had discussed the "pros" of having the PSA test, only 32% reported the doctor had discussed the "cons" of the test. Sixty per cent reported they shared the decision with their doctor, 32% said they had made the decision and 8% said the doctor had made the final decision.

The final decision will always be yours. We hope the information we have set out in the book will make that decision a much better informed one than it might otherwise have been.

Acknowledgements

We thank Prof. Alan Coates for his many detailed comments on early drafts of the book; Jessica Orchard for her proofreading; and Erin Mathieu for producing the diagrams on pages 101–02.

About the authors

Simon Chapman is professor of public health at the University of Sydney. His primary discipline is medical sociology, and within that area he has devoted his career to research and policy advocacy, being most well known for his work in tobacco control. In that field he has won numerous national and international awards, including the 2008 NSW Premier's Award for Cancer Researcher of the Year, and the 2003 American Cancer Society's Luther Terry Medal for Outstanding Individual Leadership in tobacco control. He was a board member of the Cancer Council NSW (1997–2006) and is currently a board member of Cancer Australia, the Australian government's peak advisory body on cancer control. He is a life member of the Australian Consumer's Association, and was its chairman for five years (1997–2001). One of the core principles of the consumer movement is that people should be given full and comprehensive information to help them make wise choices as consumers, including as consumers of health services like screening. He has contributed to this book in the spirit of that principle.

Alexandra Barratt is associate professor of epidemiology at the University of Sydney, where she teaches in public health, epidemiology and evidence-based medicine. Her research investigates ways to help people make more informed choices about their health care including decisions about screening for breast cancer and prostate cancer. She has produced and presented documentary radio programs for ABC Radio (*The Health Report*) on cancer screening and evidence-based medicine. She is a double Eureka prizewinner for these programs in 2006 and 2007. She has worked for the National Cancer Institute in the US, the National Breast Cancer Screening Committee in Canada, and the National Breast Cancer Centre in Australia. She sees patients at Family Planning NSW.

Martin Stockler is associate professor in cancer medicine and clinical epidemiology, consultant medical oncologist at the Sydney Cancer Centre, Royal Prince Alfred Hospital and the Concord Repatriation General Hospital, and co-director of Oncology at the National Health and Medical Research Council Clinical Trials Centre at the University of Sydney. He specialises in using drugs to treat people with cancer of the prostate, testis, kidney, bladder and related organs. His research and teaching focus on using clinical trials to improve quality and length of life, prognostication and communication for those affected by cancer.

1

What is prostate cancer and how common is it?

The prostate is an exocrine (secreting) gland in the male reproductive system. It surrounds the urethra just below the bladder and can be felt indirectly behind the rectal wall by a finger inserted into the rectum (this is known as digital rectal examination or DRE). A healthy prostate is slightly larger than a walnut. The prostate stores and secretes a milky fluid that makes up 25–30% of the semen volume, along with spermatozoa and seminal vesicle fluid. Prostatic fluid is expelled in the first ejaculate together with most of the spermatozoa.

Three main diseases can afflict the prostate: prostatitis, benign prostatic hyperplasia (BPH) and less commonly, prostate cancer.

Prostatitis is inflammation of the prostate gland. Prostatitis is a very common problem, which occurs particularly, but by no means exclusively, in older men [37]. Typical symptoms of prostatitis include fever, chills, increased urinary frequency, frequent urination at night, difficulty in urinating, burning or painful urination, pain between the anus and the scrotum (perineal pain), low-back pain, a tender or swollen prostate, blood in the urine, and painful ejaculation.

The best understood cause of prostatitis is infection with the same kinds of bacteria that cause other kinds of urinary tract infection. Acute bacterial prostatitis typically affects younger men, or those with a urinary catheter, and often causes severe symptoms. Chronic prostatitis typically affects middle-aged or older men, often causes few symptoms, and is typically found as a cause of recurrent urinary tract infections. Bacterial prostatitis is treated with antibiotics.

Chronic non-bacterial prostatitis or male chronic pelvic pain syndrome, is the diagnosis given to the 95% men who have some symptoms of prostatitis, but no evidence of bacterial infection [38]. Many treatments have been tried for this poorly understood set of symptoms, but those tested carefully, including with alpha blockers, anti-inflammatories, and alternative therapies, have shown only modest benefits at best [39].

Benign prostatic hyperplasia (BPH) occurs in older men. With ageing, the prostate often enlarges to the point where urination becomes difficult. Symptoms include needing to urinate often or delayed commencement of urination. If the prostate grows too large, it may constrict the urethra and impede the flow of urine, making urination difficult and painful, and in extreme cases completely impossible. The prostate gets larger in most men as they age. A large European study showed the prevalence of BPH is 2.7% for men aged 45–49, increasing to 24% by the age of 80 [40].

BPH can be treated with medication, a minimally invasive surgical procedure or by surgery that completely removes the prostate. Minimally invasive procedures include transurethral needle ablation of the prostate (TUNA) and transurethral microwave thermotherapy (TUMT). The surgery most often used for obstructive BPH is called transurethral resection of the prostate (TURP or TUR). In TURP, a surgical instrument is inserted into the penis through the urethra and small sections of the prostate that are pressing against the upper part of the urethra and restricting the flow of urine are shaved off from the inside, reducing the pressure on the urethra. The procedure is often colloquially known as a "rebore".

Prostate cancer is a common cancer, affecting about 20% of men by the age of 85. It is uncommon in young men (under 50) and becomes increasingly common as men age. In fact, autopsy studies show that a significant proportion of men (around 40–50%) – have prostate cancer by the age of 70. These men had no idea they had prostate cancer, so we know that prostate cancer occurs commonly and can cause no symptoms at all. Prostate cancer is the cause of death in only about 4% of men. Since it occurs in up to 50% of men, we therefore know that in many, many men it is not life threatening (see below).

Early prostate cancer causes few symptoms. In fact there are no symptoms that can differentiate prostate cancer from benign prostate diseases such as benign prostatic hyperplasia. Just like BPH it can cause problems with urination and erectile function.

Usually prostate cancer grows very slowly (see indolent cancer below) but what we call "prostate cancer" includes a spectrum of disease from slow-growing cancers through to rarer cancers that grow and spread more rapidly. Prostate cancer cells may metastasise (spread or disseminate) from the prostate to other parts of the body, such as the lymph nodes, bones, lungs and liver. Prostate cancer cells that spread to other parts of the body can cause significant symptoms, most commonly bone pain and fatigue. Prostate cancer that has spread to other parts of the body is incurable and usually fatal, but it is also treatable so that unpleasant symptoms can be reduced. Most men with metastatic prostate cancer live several or more years after it is diagnosed.

What is an "indolent" cancer?

"Indolent" means slow growing. Many may be surprised to learn that cancer can exist in the body for many years without ever becoming a problem. Thyroid cancer and lymphomas are examples of cancers which are found in people but can be indolent and non-life threatening. We know from autopsy studies that they may exist in the body for many years without causing any problems to a person. More on autopsy studies shortly.

In the past 30 years in the US, the incidence of thyroid cancer doubled while the death rate from the disease remained stable [41]. As we will see in detail later, this is also the case with prostate cancer: nearly all of this large increase in cancer incidence – 87% with thyroid cancer – can be explained by advances in diagnostic and imaging technology that enable thyroid cancer to be discovered. These developments have seen small papillary cancers being found that would have not been found with earlier diagnostic techniques. As diagnostic technology becomes more and more sophisticated and precise, evidence of disease can be found that in past times would have not come to light.

With prostate cancer, massive increases in the number of men being tested for the disease have resulted in large increases in the incidence of the disease. But just like thyroid cancer, the death rate from prostate cancer has remained remarkably stable for nearly 40 years in Australia.

Some reading this will immediately think "isn't it wonderful that advances in science have allowed us to detect these cancers earlier, so they can be treated sooner and save lives." Such thinking risks missing the point that the whole aim of medical investigation is to find and treat problems which threaten health and life. If a "problem" does neither, we need to ask why it should be thought of as a problem. The authors of the thyroid study above commented that "many of these cancers would likely never have caused symptoms during life" and the burgeoning incidence of thyroid cancer is a classic example of "overdiagnosis" [41].

Overdiagnosis means the diagnosis of conditions which would have never caused a person distressing problems of ill-health or death. It means conferring a disease label on people who are living lives untroubled by that disease and more importantly, who are unlikely to be ever troubled by that disease. Prostate cancer has been described as the *par excellence* example of overdiagnosis. This does *not* mean that there are not men whose lives are saved from early death from prostate cancer by early diagnosis. But as we shall see throughout this book, we have little way of knowing in advance *which* men will benefit from screening and which will be unnecessarily treated, often with serious adverse consequences to their life. The fundamental problem is that by screening and testing for prostate cancer we are finding many more prostate cancers than we ever did before, and strange as it may seem, many of these cancers would never become life threatening. In the past these men would never have known they had prostate cancer, they would go on to die of something else, dying *with* their prostate cancer, rather than *because of* it. By finding all these prostate cancers that are indolent we are giving many more men a prostate cancer diagnosis than ever before. Hence the term "overdiagnosis". This is the core dilemma that each man contemplating being tested faces.

What do autopsy studies show?

One way of estimating the extent of overdiagnosis in a community is via the results of autopsies carried out on people who have died while not under medical care. Autopsies are performed to determine cause of death when this has not already been established by diagnosis prior to death occurring, but can also reveal the presence of symptomless disease that was not causing the person any problems. These studies provide a unique way of estimating the prevalence of undiagnosed, often benign disease in a population. This is because people who die suddenly, while not being a random sample, nonetheless represent a wide cross-section of the population. Sudden deaths may occur more in men with dangerous occupations and who have risk factors for heart disease. These factors may introduce unknown biases that might cause the prevalence of prostate cancer to be lower or higher than in a truly random sample of the population. But the nature and direction of such biases are not obvious, and so it is likely that the picture we get from autopsy studies will provide a broadly accurate estimate of the prevalence of undetected prostate cancer in the community. Because we can compare the prevalence of symptomless prostate cancer found at autopsy with how many men develop prostatic cancer that causes symptoms and then die of it, we can get a broad estimate of the extent of overdiagnosis. In other words, autopsy studies can show us that there are some diseases which commonly don't cause symptoms at all, much less threaten life. And the prevalence of such disease is quite high.

Autopsy studies of Chinese, German, Israeli, Jamaican, Swedish, and Ugandan men who died of other causes (such as sudden death through injury, homicide, suicide or heart attack) have found prostate cancer in 10–20% of men in their 50s, and in a remarkable 40–50% of men in their 70s [42]. In a Pittsburgh (US) study of 340 sudden death victims who had donated their organs for transplantation, it was found that across all age groups combined, 12% of men had prostate cancer. From age 40, the proportion of men with evidence of the disease began to rise. Among men aged 50–59, 23% had incidental prostate cancer and among those aged 60–69, 35% (approximately one in three) had incidental prostate cancer. In the oldest group (aged 70–81) 46% of men were harbouring the disease [43].

These studies provide a unique way of estimating the prevalence of undiagnosed, often benign disease in a population. The take-home message from these studies is that benign, symptomless prostate cancer is very common in men, especially in later life. Men live without knowing they have the disease and most will never be affected adversely by it, dying of some other cause with "silent" prostate cancer having been in their bodies for many years. As prostate cancer did not kill these men, it is clear that finding and treating their prostate cancer would not have delivered any health benefit, nor extended their lives.

2

What is the risk of dying from prostate cancer?

We will all one day die of some cause that will be entered on our death certificate by our doctor or determined by a coroner if we have died suddenly without having been under recent medical care. In 2007, 70,569 men died in Australia out of a total male population of 10,358,791, meaning that 0.68% of men – around one in 147 – died in that year from *any* cause. Table 1 shows numbers and percentages of total deaths for the top 20 causes of death in males.

Table 1: Leading underlying specific causes of male death, all ages, 2007

Rank	Cause of death	Number of deaths	% all male deaths
1	Coronary heart diseases	12,119	17.2
2	Lung cancer	4715	6.7
3	Cerebrovascular diseases	4516	6.4
4	Chronic obstructive pulmonary disease	2965	4.2
5	Prostate cancer	2938	4.2
6	Dementia and Alzheimer's disease	2415	3.4
7	Colorectal cancer	2221	3.1
8	Diabetes	1923	2.7
9	Unknown primary site cancers	1832	2.6

Rank	Cause of death	Number of deaths	% all male deaths
10	Suicide	1453	2.1
11	Heart failure and complications and ill-defined heart diseases	1361	1.9
12	Pancreatic cancer	1233	1.7
13	Kidney failure	1163	1.6
14	Influenza and pneumonia	1160	1.6
15	Liver diseases	977	1.4
16	Land transport accidents	948	1.3
17	Leukaemia	892	1.3
18	Melanoma	864	1.2
19	Oesophageal cancer	790	1.1
20	Lymphomas	780	1.1
	All deaths	70,569	100.0

Source: Australian Institute of Health and Welfare National Mortality Database.

But what about prostate cancer as a cause of cancer death? Table 2 below showing cancer incidence and death indicates that prostate cancer is the second highest cause of *cancer* death in men in Australia after lung cancer. With 2938 deaths out of 70,569 male deaths in 2007, about 4.2% of all men's deaths across all ages in that year were from prostate cancer. The probability of any given male of any age dying of prostate cancer *in a single year* was 0.03% or one in 3513. But as we will show below, this proportion is far larger for men in older age groups, because deaths from prostate cancer are very rare in men aged less than 40 and very uncommon in men aged less than 50. Men aged over 50 are sometimes described as being "at risk" for prostate cancer, although some urologists have recently tried to widen that label to include men in their 40s (see p43).

Table 2: New cases (incidence) of selected common cancers in males (2006) and mortality (2007) from those cancers, Australia

	New cases (incidence)			
Cancer site/ type	Number	Per cent of total cancer	Crude rate per 100,000	Risk to age 85
Prostate	17,444	29.5	170.0	1 in 5
Colon	4566	7.7	45.9	1 in 16
Melanoma	6051	10.2	59.6	1 in 14
Lung, bronchus & trachea	6030	10.2	60.6	1 in 12
Rectum	2866	4.9	28.3	1 in 27
Lymphoma	2518	4.3	24.7	1 in 33
Head and neck	2059	3.5	19.9	1 in 40
Bladder	1764	3.0	18.1	1 in 38
Kidney	1625	2.8	15.9	1 in 51
Leukaemia	1513	2.6	15.2	1 in 52
Stomach	1277	2.2	12.9	1 in 55
Pancreas	1158	2.1	10.2	1 in 70
All cancers	59,058	100.0	584.6	1 in 2

	Deaths		
	Number	Per cent of total deaths	Mean age at death
Lung, bronchus & trachea	4715	6.7	72.0
Prostate	2938	4.2	79.8
Colon	1295	1.8	73.0
Pancreas	1233	1.7	70.7
Rectum	896	1.3	70.6
Leukaemia	892	1.3	71.7

	Deaths		
	Number	Per cent of total deaths	Mean age at death
Melanoma	864	1.2	69.2
Oesophagus	790	1.1	69.3
Lymphoma	780	1.1	71.9
Stomach	704	1.0	71.6
Head and neck	667	0.9	68.3
All cancer except prostate	19,624	27.8	71.5
All cancers	22,562	32.0	72.6

Sources: www.aihw.gov.au/cancer/index.cfm and correspondence from AIHW dated 26 July 2010.

As we saw above, the risk of a man dying of prostate cancer *in one year* was a very low 0.03% or one in 3513, and about 4% of all men will die from prostate cancer. Mostly these deaths occur at advanced ages. A man's chance of dying of prostate cancer increases with age. Table 3 shows the numbers, rates per 100,000 men and probabilities of death of prostate cancer in one year in Australia.

As can be seen in the first column of Table 3, of the 2938 men who died from prostate cancer in 2007, more than half (1716 or 58%) were aged 80 or over and 82% were aged 70 or more. Just 2.8% (83 men) were aged less than 60, and 10 (0.1%) were in their 40s. The average age of death (note that this is a different concept than "life expectancy") in men in Australia in 2007 was 76 years (see Table 2). So men who die from any cause after that time are already living longer than average. The data in the US are remarkably similar. There, the median age of death from prostate cancer from 2000 through to 2004 was 80 years, and 71% of deaths occurred in men older than

75 years [13]. These figures will surprise many men accustomed to reading about men of much younger age dying of prostate cancer. Some certainly do die in middle age, but compared with death rates from other cancers, relatively fewer men die from prostate cancer in middle age.

Table 3: Number and rate of prostate cancer deaths and probability of death in one year, Australia 2007

Age group and number of prostate cancer deaths	Rate per 100,000 and probability of death in one year
40–44#: 3	0.4 (1 in 250,000)
45–49: 7	0.9 (1 in 111,111)
50–54: 18	2.6 (1 in 38,462)
55–59: 55	8.7 (1 in 11,494)
60–64: 142	26.6 (1 in 3759)
65–69: 215	53.8 (1 in 1859)
70–74: 315	101.1 (1 in 989)
75–79: 567	223.1 (1 in 448)
80–84: 713	413.8 (1 in 242)
85+: 903	800.9 (1 in 125)
All ages: 2938	31.0 (1 in 3226)

Source: www.aihw.gov.au/cancer/data/acim_books/index.cfm (prostate cancer)
no deaths were recorded in men less than 40

What are the historic trends in prostate cancer deaths in Australia?

The total *number* of men dying in Australia from prostate cancer is increasing slowly each year. In the 39 years between 1968 and 2007, prostate cancer deaths grew from 963 to 2938, an average annual increase of 51 deaths per year, or one a week [44]. The two main reasons for this growth are that the age structure of the population is changing and the size of the population is growing. We have an aging population in Australia (the proportion of the total population in older age groups is steadily increasing). So both the number and the proportion of older people in the community are increasing as the post-World War II baby-boomer generation grows into old age. Moreover, because we have been so successful in reducing deaths from many causes of death that in past decades would have killed people earlier in life, many more men are surviving longer and so the numbers and proportions of deaths caused by diseases like cancer which tend to kill people later in life are rising. Life expectancy has increased. In 1950, male life expectancy in Australia was only 66.5. Today's 79 years is a remarkable 18.8% increase on that, all in what is less than an eye blink of time in human history.

Major causes of death in men such as lung cancer, heart disease and motor vehicle injury have decreased dramatically in this period too. Because people have to die of some cause, reductions in some causes of death inevitably mean that more men will die from other causes instead. For example, if we want to see the rates per 100,000 of lung cancer deaths we see today in men, we have to travel back to 1962 [45].

However, by looking at the age-standardised death rate per 100,000 men over time we get a very different picture, helpful in thinking about the question of whether this disease is really claiming "more" lives today. Age-standardised rates adjust for any changes in the age distribution in the population over time and so allow a valid comparison of rates over time. Table 4 is worth studying closely. Several broad trends are obvious. First, in the 39 years 1968–2007, the age-standardised death *rate* from prostate cancer has varied very little, with an average of 35.8 per 100,000 men and a range of 32.2 to 43.7. The most recent rate in 2007 (31 per 100,000) was very similar to the death rate at the beginning of this 38-year series in 1968 (35.6/100,000). In between there was a rise in the death rate (in the early- to mid-1990s) which has now reversed back to rates seen in the early 1970s, a decade before the PSA test became available. ("Incidence" means the number of new cases of prostate cancer diagnosed in that year).

However, looking at the data on cancer *incidence*, the same basically flat trend we see for deaths is not apparent. Instead we see a dramatic leap in the incidence of the disease from the early 1990s. This change has been largely sustained ever since, resulting in a startling difference in the risk of men being diagnosed with prostate cancer before the 1990s (approximately one in 22 men in their lifetime) to nearly three times that today (one in eight).

These patterns are obvious in Figure 1 below.

Two obvious questions arise here: what has caused this massive increase in the incidence of the disease? And if the death rates from the disease today are almost the same as they were 38 years ago when the known incidence of the disease was much lower, then what can be said about the relationship between the rising incidence of the disease and the failure of the death rate to change in the same dramatic fashion?

Table 4: Age-standardised death and incidence rates of prostate cancer, 1968–2006

Year	Death rate per 100,000	Risk to age 75 of death from prostate cancer	Incidence rate per 100,000	Risk to age 75 of prostate cancer being diagnosed
1968	35.6	1 in 78	National incidence data were not kept prior to 1982 in Australia	
1969	33.4	1 in 77		
1970	36.8	1 in 74		
1971	32.6	1 in 84		
1972	32.4	1 in 78		
1973	34.1	1 in 70		
1974	33.2	1 in 77		
1975	34.3	1 in 83		
1976	33.0	1 in 72		
1977	34.0	1 in 78		
1978	32.2	1 in 82		
1979	33.6	1 in 72		
1980	33.4	1 in 76		
1981	33.4	1 in 79		
1982	34.5	1 in 77	80.8	1 in 23
1983	34.7	1 in 82	80.1	1 in 24
1984	33.3	1 in 73	83.2	1 in 22
1985	35.7	1 in 80	82.9	1 in 22
1986	35.7	1 in 72	85.5	1 in 22
1987	37.2	1 in 73	85.7	1 in 22
1988	37.6	1 in 66	92.7	1 in 21

Year	Death rate per 100,000	Risk to age 75 of death from prostate cancer	Incidence rate per 100,000	Risk to age 75 of prostate cancer being diagnosed
1989	39.6	1 in 68	102.7	1 in 20
1990	39.7	1 in 65	110.1	1 in 17
1991	39.3	1 in 68	124.1	1 in 16
1992	41.2	1 in 60	165.0	1 in 14
1993	43.7	1 in 62	184.2	1 in 9
1994	43.6	1 in 63	168.6	1 in 8
1995	41.2	1 in 63	137.6	1 in 8
1996	41.3	1 in 68	129.9	1 in 10
1997	36.8	1 in 74	128.0	1 in 11
1998	37.2	1 in 74	129.7	1 in 11
1999	35.2	1 in 82	128.4	1 in 11
2000	35.9	1 in 76	130.6	1 in 11
2001	35.2	1 in 82	134.5	1 in 11
2002	35.3	1 in 84	147.2	1 in 10
2003	34.5	1 in 80	164.3	1 in 9
2004	32.9	1 in 88	164.4	1 in 8
2005	33.5	1 in 86	166.6	1 in 8
2006	32.3	1 in 89	170.0	1 in 7
2007	31.0	1 in 104	Not available	

Source: www.aihw.gov.au/cancer/index.cfm (cancer incidence and mortality data)

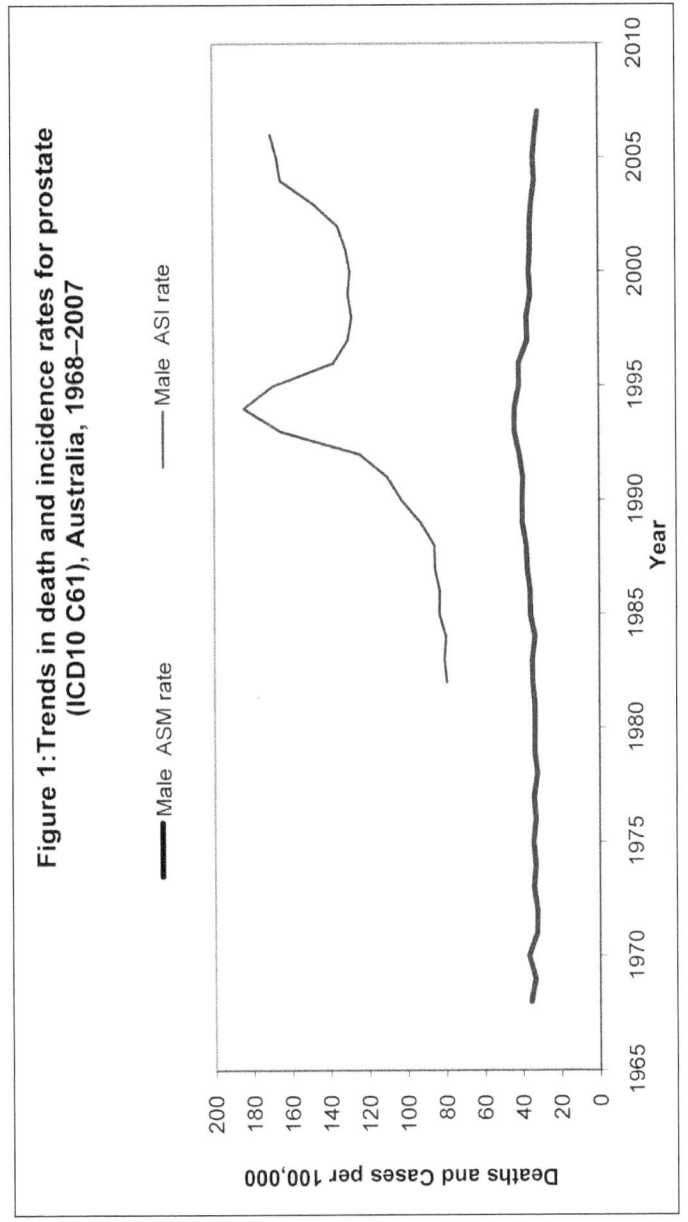

Figure 1: Trends in death and incidence rates for prostate (ICD10 C61), Australia, 1968–2007

Source: Age-standardised to the Australian Standard Population 2001. Australian Institute of Health and Welfare (AIHW) 2010. ACIM (Australian Cancer Incidence and Mortality) Books. AIHW: Canberra

The answer to the first question is simple: we are finding more cancers because there is more testing. The rising incidence of the disease does *not* mean that within a few years, there was somehow a sudden "spread" or rise of the disease – that many more Australian men were somehow acquiring prostate cancer. There is no claim being made by anyone that this has occurred, in the way for example we can easily demonstrate historical rises in the incidence of lung cancer as a time-lagged response to rising smoking rates 30 to 40 years before. Instead, the rise can be readily explained by the spread of PSA testing and the related phenomenon of the rise of voices urging that men be screened for the disease.

The second question – why there has been no significant change to the prostate cancer death rate in nearly 40 years – suggests that if the main argument in favour of finding all the previously undiagnosed prostate cancer is that this will reduce deaths from the disease, then this plainly has *not* happened. Further evidence relevant to this fundamental point is discussed on page 97 where we consider the results of two important randomised controlled trials of the PSA test, examining whether screening across a large number of men saves lives.

3

What is the risk of being diagnosed with prostate cancer?

Just as the risk of dying from prostate cancer increases as Men age, so does the risk of being diagnosed with prostate cancer (i.e. its incidence). This is clear in Figure 2 below, which shows that prostate cancer is very rare in men under 40 but rises steadily with age from around the age of 40 to around the age of 70 when the incidence curve flattens out.

Advancing age is the most important risk factor for death from nearly every disease. Except for certain illnesses of infancy and childhood, and road deaths (which peak in people in their 20s), nearly every cause of death is far more common in older than younger people. The same is very true for prostate cancer. In Table 2, we saw that the average age that men died from prostate cancer in Australian in 2007 was 79.8, quite easily the oldest average age from death from any of the major causes of cancer death shown. All the other causes of cancer death kill men on average some seven to eleven years earlier. Table 5 shows both the number of men diagnosed in 2005 in each age group, and the age-specific rate of prostate cancer diagnosis per 100,000 men in each age group.

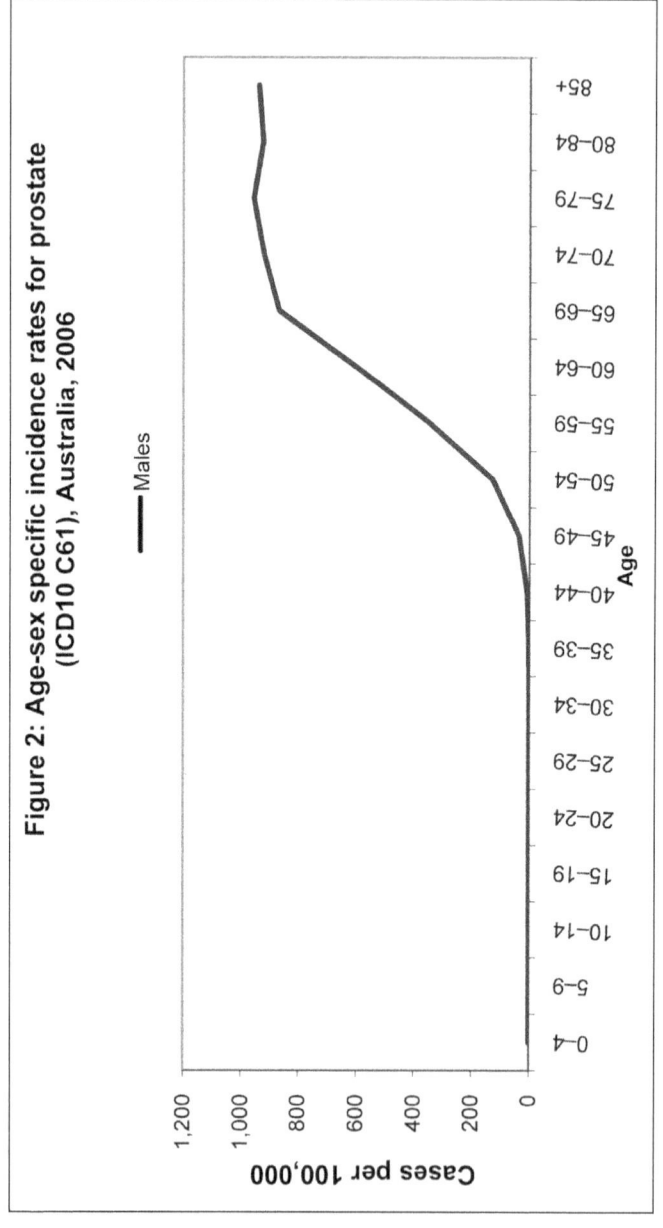

Figure 2: Age-sex specific incidence rates for prostate (ICD10 C61), Australia, 2006

Source: Australian Institute of Health and Welfare (AIHW) 2010. ACIM (Australian Cancer Incidence and Mortality) Books. AIHW: Canberra

Of the 17,444 cases of prostate cancer diagnosed in 2006, just 329 (1.9%) occurred in men aged less than 50. By contrast, 11,079 (63.5%) were in men aged 65 and over. Adjusted for the number of men in each age band, Table 5 shows that the likelihood of a man aged 75–79 (where the odds are highest) being diagnosed as having prostate cancer in one year is one in 232, some 227 times more likely than a man aged 40–44, where the disease is uncommon, and 4274 times more than a man aged 30–34, where the disease is extremely rare. The probabilities of any man aged less than 40 being diagnosed with prostate cancer are thus *far* lower than those of winning first prize in a lottery where 200,000 tickets are typically sold. These are astronomically low odds. The rate at which men aged 40–44 are being diagnosed with prostate cancer is one in 52,632 and from age 45–49, one in 6,250 – still a very low risk.

Table 5: Number and rate of prostate cancer diagnoses, different age groups, Australia 2005.

Age-group and number of prostate cancer diagnoses	Rate per 100,000 men	Age-group and number of prostate cancer diagnoses	Rate per 100,000 men
20–24: 1	0.1 (1 in 1 million)	55–59: 2037	164.5 (1 in 608)
25–29: 0	0 (–)	60–64: 2572	274.5 (1 in 364)
30–34: 1	0.1 (1 in 1 million)	65–69: 3141	412.0 (1 in 243)
35–39: 3	0.2 (1 in 500,000)	70–74: 2672	427.0 (1 in 234)
40–44: 29	1.9 (1 in 52,632)	75–79: 2372	431.9 (1 in 232)
45–49: 235	16.0 (1 in 6250)	80–84: 1474	372.5 (1 in 268)
50–54: 803	60.0 (1 in 1667)	85+: 988	323.8 (1 in 309)

Source: d01.aihw.gov.au/cognos/cgi-bin/ppdscgi.exe?DC=Q&E=/Cancer/australia_age_specific_1982_2005

Yet in 2010, the Prostate Cancer Foundation of Australia ran TV advertising featuring several Australian male sporting and acting celebrities in their 30s saying to camera that every year prostate cancer kills men "just like me". As we saw in Table 2, in 2007 there were no cases of men "just like them" in their 30s who died of prostate cancer in Australia. Many young men seeing these advertisements with the rapid cavalcade of highly recognisable men in their 30s and 40s, would assume that it was common for men of this age to die of prostate cancer. This is a highly misleading message.

The chance of having prostate cancer diagnosed depends not only on age but on the extent to which men voluntarily come forward to be tested to see if they have the disease. What we know is that the more we look for prostate cancer, the more we will find. So the lifetime odds of a man being diagnosed depend very strongly on the extent to which men come forward to be tested. If few come forward, far fewer will be diagnosed and so the probability of any man in the community getting a diagnosis will be lower.

As we saw before, if a man was to conscientiously get PSA tested every year from (say) age 50, we know from autopsy studies that about 12% of men in their 40s, and around 40% of men in their 70s [42] could be found to have the disease, if only we looked carefully enough for it. There is a huge reservoir of prostate cancer in the community that could be found if we test enough people, often enough. If those promoting testing are successful, many more men could be diagnosed with prostate cancer and thereafter have to live with this knowledge. Many would undergo traumatic surgical intervention which may profoundly affect their lives. But because the death rates from prostate cancer have barely changed in nearly 40 years, what would have been the point in all this early disease finding?

In 2009, the Urological Society of Australia called for all men in their 40s (and over) to get themselves tested. So far, no group of urologists or prostate screening advocates have called for men *under* 40 to be screened, but by the same "finding a needle in a haystack" reasoning behind the call to screen 40–50-year olds, it may not be inconceivable that someone will reduce the recommended testing age even lower.

By spreading concern and some anxiety to men in their 40s about the disease, a large number might get tested, to the obvious financial benefit of the diagnostic industries concerned. As we will see later in the book (see p81) such testing will result in a large number of men having their prostates surgically removed, and a significant proportion of these men having serious and lasting side effects of that surgery such as sexual impotence.

Why are we seeing increases in prostate cancer in Australia?

Today, after non-melanoma forms of skin cancer, prostate cancer is easily the most commonly diagnosed cancer in Australia. As can readily be seen in Table 6, since 1988 there have been a series of dramatic increases in the number of newly diagnosed cases of prostate cancer in Australia, most particularly between 1988 and 1994, and 2002–2004. The 41% leap in cases between 1992 and 1993 was unprecedented. On the surface, some people would be tempted to look at this data and assume there has been a growing epidemic of prostate cancer in Australia.

However, Australia's experience mirrors that of many countries where the incidence of prostate cancer diagnosis rose after the introduction and promotion of the Prostate Specific Antigen (PSA) test in 1987–88. No-one knowledgeable about cancer would argue that these rapid rising numbers means that the "actual" incidence of prostate cancer is rising: it is not like the growth of obesity in recent decades. There is not actually more prostate cancer in the community. What the rises mean is simply that *more* men are being tested and because of this, more cancer is being found.

Table 6: New cases of prostate cancer, Australia 1982–2005 (percentage change from previous year)

1982: 3680	1995: 12369 (–5.4)
1983: 3744 (+1.7)	1996: 10304 (–16.7)
1984: 3884 (+3.7)	1997: 9993 (–3.0)
1985: 4156 (+7)	1998: 10087 (+1.1)
1986: 4306 (+3.6)	1999: 10581 (+4.9)
1987: 4563 (+6)	2000: 10835 (+2.4)
1988: 4767 (+4.5)	2001: 11389 (+5.1)
1989: 5301 (+11.2)	2002: 12177 (+6.9)
1990: 6109 (+15.2)	2003: 13774 (+12.9)
1991: 6755 (+10.6)	2004: 15898 (+15.4)
1992: 7920 (+17.2)	2005: 16560 (+4.2)
1993: 11180 (+41.2)	2006: 17444 (+13.5)
1994: 13073 (+16.9)	

Sources: d01.aihw.gov.au/cognos/cgi-bin/ppdscgi.exe?DC=Q&E=/Cancer/australia_age_specific_1982_2005 and www.aihw.gov.au/cancer/data/acim_books/index.cfm

What are Australian men told about prostate cancer in the media?

Prostate cancer has become a big health news story, being the third most reported cancer after breast cancer and melanoma [46]. Much of this reportage – although certainly not all – is accurate and important in raising awareness [47]. But overwhelmingly, it actively promotes screening. As we saw at the beginning of this book, even though nearly all expert bodies which have reviewed the evidence on the ability of screening to save lives have concluded that the risks outweigh the benefits and that the number of lives saved because of screening would be small, this is decidedly not the message that is being communicated to men in the media [48].

In a study one of us (SC) published in 2007 on the accuracy of media reports about prostate cancer in 388 Australian newspaper and 42 television items, one in ten statements reported to the public were found to be inaccurate [47]. Examples of these included:

Prostate cancer, which kills more men in this country than any other form of the disease

Prostate cancer is ... the biggest cause of cancer death in males ... treat men for their commonest lethal cancer [wrong! Lung cancer kills far more]

Prostate cancer is the second biggest killer of Australian men [wrong! Heart disease, lung cancer, stroke and chronic obstructive pulmonary disease kill more men].

As we finished writing this book in August 2010, the Prostate Cancer Foundation of Australia's website [49] states, "Each year in Australia, close to 3,300 men die of prostate cancer – equal to the number of women who die from breast cancer annually." In fact, there has never been a year in which "close to 3,300" men died of prostate cancer in Australia. The highest number that has ever occurred in one year was in 2005, when 2950 men died from the disease. In 2008, the Australian Institute of Health and Welfare (AIHW) published a projection for the number of prostate cancer deaths in Australia of 3366 in 2010 [50]. In the same report, it projected the figure of 3124 deaths from the disease in 2007. But in fact, as we saw in Table 1, 2938 men died from the disease in 2007 (the latest year for which data is available) – some 6% less than projected. The "3,330 each year" figure is therefore nearly 13% higher than the highest number ever recorded.

The Foundation's chief executive, Andrew Giles, was reported in *The Sydney Morning Herald* in July 2010 as claiming that prostate cancer would soon become the No. 1 killer of Australian men:

> By about 2015 the number of men this disease is killing is going to exceed the number of men who die of lung cancer, because that tumour is coming down thanks to all the work we do in tobacco control. So prostate cancer will be the number one killer of men. [51]

So how credible is this claim? In December 2008, AIHW estimated that in 2010 there would be 4687 deaths from lung cancer and 3366 deaths from prostate cancer [50]. In fact, in 2007 – the latest available year, there were 4715 lung cancer deaths and 2938 deaths from prostate cancer. Far from going down, lung cancer deaths averaged 4675 across the seven years (2001–07). In the three years between 2007 and 2010, the AIHW estimated that deaths from prostate cancer would grow by 428, or an average of 143 deaths a year. If this continued until 2015, this would mean that in the seven years (2007–2015), an extra 1000 deaths per year might occur, giving a rough total of 3939. If total lung cancer deaths continue to plateau as they have between 2006 and 2010, this would mean that Mr Giles' prediction would fall some 746 deaths short – about a 25% overestimate.

In 2007, Professor John Shine, head of Sydney's Garvan Institute, sent a fundraising letter to thousands of potential donors. It stated, "every single hour at least one man dies of prostate cancer". Author (SC) wrote to the Garvan pointing out that this statement was massively incorrect. If prostate cancer killed one man an hour there would be 8760 deaths from the disease each year in Australia. With 2952 deaths in 2006, they overstated the true figure by 5808 – nearly 300% – explained later as an error arising from an extrapolation from UK data, unadjusted from that nation's far greater population.

On 5 June 2007, Dr Andrew Rochford from Channel 7's *What's Good for You* stated that "prostate cancer is second only to heart disease" in killing Australian men. Prostate cancer is not "second only to heart disease" as a cause of death either. Prostate cancer was in fact the sixth leading cause of death in men, a very long way behind ischemic heart disease which kills 13,152 men a year; stroke (4826); lung cancer (4733); other heart disease (3290); and chronic obstructive pulmonary disease (2986). Further, ischemic heart disease causes much more disability in the community than prostate cancer. Ischemic heart disease causes the loss of 151,107 DALYs (Disability Adjusted Life Years), compared with 36,546 lost to prostate cancer, putting it in ninth place by that criterion.

In August 2010, the Prostate Cancer Foundation issued press releases to publicise a conference it was hosting in Queensland. One report stated "the National Cancer Institute in the USA has in the last month reversed previous opposition to PSA tests and thrown out previous contrary studies". We wrote to the NCI to ask whether this statement was accurate. They replied saying "Please note that as a Federal research agency, the NCI does not set screening guidelines". They also referred us to the website of the Agency for Healthcare Research and Quality (AHRQ) which they said

> is the Federal agency responsible for setting screening guidelines. You may wish to explore the U.S. Preventive Services Task Force (USPSTF) "Screening for Prostate Cancer: Recommendation Statement."

The USPSTF, which is sponsored by the AHRQ, is an independent panel of experts in primary care and prevention that rigorously evaluates clinical research in order to assess the merits of preventive measures, including screening tests. The link provided (www.uspreventiveservicestaskforce.org/uspstf/uspsprca.htm) states unequivocally:

> The USPSTF concludes that the current evidence is insufficient to assess the balance of benefits and harms of prostate cancer screening in men younger than age 75 years.
>
> The USPSTF recommends against screening for prostate cancer in men age 75 years or older.

In other words, the idea that the NCI was ever "opposed" to prostate screening is misleading, as is the idea that the NCI has now "reversed" such opposition.

These examples are a small taste of some of the misinformation that is circulating about prostate cancer.

4

What increases or decreases the risk of prostate cancer?

Does prostate cancer "run in families"? If you have relatives who have had prostate cancer, are your chances higher of getting the disease?

Increasing age is the strongest predictor of a diagnosis of prostate cancer, but the second most important predictor is family history. Around 10–20% of men with prostate cancer have a family history of the disease (meaning that 80–90% don't) [52]. Given what we have summarised earlier about many men dying *with* rather than *from* prostate cancer, and never knowing that they had the disease, it is possible that part of this apparent excess rate in men with a family history may be due to their higher participation in testing. We know of no studies that have considered this possibility. Men who have a first degree relative (a father or brother) who has had prostate cancer are twice as likely to be diagnosed with prostate cancer as men with no affected relative [53]. The risk increases with the increasing number of affected relatives and with decreasing age at the diagnosis of those with the disease. Men with family history of prostate cancer typically have the disease diagnosed six to seven years earlier than men without a family history [52]. This can often be due to increased concern about the disease in such men and their willingness to be regularly tested [54].

The most recent and largest meta-analysis on family history and prostate cancer (a meta-analysis is a study which combines all published high quality studies about a topic to assess what they all say when combined together) found the following increased risks [55]. In summary, cancer risk increases with:

1. Earlier onset of the disease in other family members
2. Increased total number of affected relatives in the family
3. Increased number of first degree relatives affected by the disease. [54]

Table 7: Family history and the probability of prostate cancer diagnosis

Relatives with prostate cancer	Relative risk (95% confidence interval)
One First degree relative (FDR)	2.57 (2.32–2.84)
Brother only	3.37 (2.07–3.83)
Father only	2.17 (1.90–2.49)
Two or more FDRs	5.08 (3.31–7.79)
One FDR diagnosed younger than 65 years	2.47 (1.71–3.55)
One FDR diagnosed older than 65 years	1.72 (1.41–2.10)

Note: A relative risk (RR) of 1 means that there would be no difference for the probability of a prostate cancer diagnosis between a man with a family history of the disease and a man with no such history. A RR of 2.57 thus means that a man with the family history has 2.57 times the likelihood of such a diagnosis compared to a man with no such history.

Unfortunately, a reliable genetic test that can discriminate between men at risk and not at risk is currently unavailable [56].

The 2010 Prostate Cancer Foundation advertising campaign gave this message to men: all men over 50 should consult their doctor about being tested, and that all men between 40 and 50 with a "family history" of the disease should also consult their doctor. As we saw earlier, the great majority of prostate cancer diagnoses and deaths occur in older men. It follows from this that the great majority of men with a relative with a family history will have had those relatives diagnosed and/or die with prostate cancer late in life.

As stated above, the risk of being diagnosed with prostate cancer is increased by a factor of about two to three if your father had prostate cancer. For a man in his early 40s, this increases his risk of being diagnosed with prostate cancer from about one in 52,000 to about one in 17,000 to 26,000; for a man in his early 50s, it would increase the risk from about one in 1600 to about one in 500 to 800 (see Table 5).

Some who advocate PSA screening in younger men argue that prostate cancer is more aggressive when it is diagnosed in younger men. Recent, detailed studies have had conflicting results, some suggesting that prostate cancer diagnosed in younger men is more aggressive than average, others suggesting it is less aggressive [57, 58]. The outcomes of prostate cancer treatment in younger men are probably as good or better than those in older men. However, there is no doubt that men diagnosed with prostate cancer at a younger age have more at stake: their average life expectancy without prostate cancer is longer; left untreated, the prostate cancer has more time to cause further problems; if treated, the prostate cancer has more time to recur.

Can anything be done to prevent prostate cancer?

With some cancers, we know that avoidance of particular exposures (ultra-violet radiation from sunlight and solaria, radiation, smoking, asbestos, soil radon, certain industrial chemicals) can do much to reduce the risk of getting cancer. So what is the situation with preventing prostate cancer?

Diet

Dietary factors are associated with both the promotion and protection of many diseases and health-related conditions: some types of diet promote some cancers and others appear to protect against some cancers [59]. Different diets are associated with both a higher and lower prevalence of various diseases and there is growing community understanding of this broad principle. Indeed, in a recent study, 73% of Australian men who had a family history of prostate cancer believed that diet was a factor associated with prostate cancer [60]. So are there *in fact* diets which appear to be associated with a lower population incidence of prostate cancer?

If you search Google for "diet and prostate cancer" you will get 2,240,000 hits. The great majority of these are entrepreneurial complementary (alternative) medicine sites promoting and selling a large range of dietary supplements, most of which will probably do little but generate expensive urine for you. There is unfortunately little accepted scientific evidence that dietary modification (reducing or increasing the intake of certain foods or elements) is a reliable way of reducing the risk of acquiring prostate cancer. Below we summarise some of the more important systematic reviews and large trials in the accumulated evidence about whether this disease can be prevented.

Overall diet

A recently published report from Victoria, a multicultural state where one can find a diversity of diets, followed 14,627 men aged 34 to 75 years for an average of 13.6 years, and identified 1018 cases of prostate cancer in the study group. The study "found no association between any dietary pattern and prostate cancer risk overall" nor did it find any association with cancer aggressiveness, Gleason score (see p67) or age at diagnosis [61].

Green tea

Daily consumption of green tea has long been thought to have a protective effect on cancer. A July 2009 Cochrane review of the role of green tea consumption in reducing the incidence of cancer (including prostate cancer) involved 51 studies with more than 1.6 million participants. The review concluded that

> The evidence that the consumption of green tea might reduce the risk of cancer was conflicting. This means that drinking green tea remains unproven in cancer prevention, but appears to be safe at moderate, regular and habitual use. [62]

Lycopene (tomatoes)

In the US in particular, it has become common for men to try to regularly eat tomatoes because of beliefs that their high content of lycopene – an anti-oxidant – may protect against prostate cancer. An analysis of 19 published studies on this subject concluded

> our results show that tomato products may play a role in the prevention of prostate cancer. However, this effect is modest. Despite the preventive benefits of lycopene found in this study, the existing evidence is not overwhelming enough to recommend the use of lycopene supplements in the prevention of prostate cancer.

The only benefit – which was statistically small – was seen in those who ate high amounts of tomato [63].

Selenium and vitamin E

A large double-blinded trial of either and both selenium and vitamin E undertaken among 35,533 men recruited in 427 North American sites where the median follow-up period was 5.46 years showed that selenium (a trace mineral) or vitamin E, alone or in combination did not prevent prostate cancer in this population of relatively healthy men compared with placebo [64].

Chemoprevention (finasteride)

Finasteride is a drug which inhibits the action of 5a-reductase, the enzyme that converts testosterone to the more potent androgen dihydrotestosterone. It is used to treat benign prostatic hyperplasia or BPH (see p22) and is also used by millions of men around the world to control baldness. The development of finasteride also allowed the possibility of studies being conducted to see if lowering androgen levels in the prostate would reduce the risk of prostate cancer. The Prostate Cancer Prevention Trial [65] set out to test this hypothesis. It involved allocating

> 18,882 men aged 55 years and over who had normal digital rectal examinations and a PSA level of 3.0 ng per millilitre or lower to treatment with finasteride (5 mg per day) or placebo for seven years. Prostate biopsy was recommended if during the trial, the annual PSA level, adjusted for the effect of finasteride, exceeded 4.0 ng per millilitre or if the digital rectal examination was abnormal.

The study directors calculated that

> 60 per cent of participants would have prostate cancer diagnosed during the study or would undergo biopsy at the end of the study and the main outcome of interest was the prevalence of prostate cancer during the seven years of the study.

The study demonstrated that by taking this drug every day for seven years, 18.4% of the men on finasteride developed prostate cancer compared with 24.4% of men on the placebo, a relative reduction of 24.8% in prevalence over the seven-year period.

However, adverse sexual side effects were more common in the finasteride-treated men: reduced ejaculatory volume 60.4% in finasteride group vs 47.3% in control group; erectile dysfunction (67.4% vs 61.5%); loss of libido (65.4% vs 59.6%); gynecomastia (developing "man boobs", 4.5% vs 2.8%). In addition, aggressive tumours of Gleason grade 7, 8, 9, or 10 were more common in the finasteride group (37%) than in the placebo group (22.2%). The study authors concluded that the drug

> prevents or delays the appearance of prostate cancer, but this possible benefit ... must be weighed against sexual side effects and the increased risk of high-grade prostate cancer.

By saying it "prevents", they of course do not mean that it prevents the disease in all men taking it, but that it reduces the incidence of the disease. And the absolute size of this reduction was only 6% – 24.4% of men not taking the drug for seven years were diagnosed with prostate cancer, while 18.4% of the men on finasteride developed prostate cancer. Moreover and very tellingly,

> there was no significant difference in the number of deaths between the two groups: five men in each group died from prostate cancer.

Subsequently, further analyses of this trial have suggested that there may not have been an increased risk of more aggressive cancers in the finasteride group after all [66, 67]. It is possible that this apparent increase was caused by biases in reporting the results of biopsies among men in the finasteride group. Analyses adjusting for this bias found little or no increased risk of high grade cancer with finasteride; in fact finasteride may even reduce the risk of developing aggressive prostate cancer, just as it appears to reduce the risk of prostate cancer overall.

So to summarise, we have good evidence that finasteride produces a modest reduction in prostate cancer with long term use. But those taking it have elevated levels of sexual problems. That information should be entered into men's calculations when deciding whether to take it.

Ejaculatory frequency

Because the prostate is a sexual organ which supplies fluid to the ejaculate, it is understandable that researchers have considered the possibility that frequency of ejaculation (high, low, and at what stages in life) might have something to do with prostate cancer. Studies have produced mixed findings. A large cohort study of 29,342 US health professional men found that

> Most categories of ejaculation frequency were unrelated to risk of prostate cancer. However, high ejaculation frequency was related to decreased risk of total prostate cancer.

Averaged across their lifetime, men who reported 21 or more ejaculations per month compared with men reporting four to seven ejaculations per month had a reduced relative risk of prostate cancer of 0.67 (95% CI, 0.51–0.89) – in other words, a 33% reduced risk. Other than for this high frequency category of ejaculation, the authors concluded, "Our results suggest that ejaculation frequency is not related to increased risk of prostate cancer" [68]. However, a more recent study showed that men who engaged in frequent masturbation, of about two to seven times a week, during their 20s and 30s, had a higher rate of prostate cancer, while men who engaged in masturbation once a week during their 50s had a lower rate [69].

These studies do not really provide men with much confidence to embark on a changed ejaculatory regimen, justifying it with hopes of preventing prostate cancer.

Physical activity

A 2001 review of the published literature on whether being physically active might protect against prostate cancer found that the "epidemiologic data supporting this hypothesis are weak and inconsistent" [70]. But of course physical activity is to be recommended for its many other important health promoting effects, including the prevention of other types of cancer.

5

How is prostate cancer diagnosed?

The Prostate Specific Antigen (PSA) test first became available in 1987 and began to be widely used and promoted thereafter. The test is done by obtaining a blood sample which is then sent to a pathology laboratory for analysis. The test measures the level of Prostate Specific Antigen in the blood. Prostate Specific Antigen is a protein made mainly in the prostate gland and low levels of PSA are normally present in the blood. As a man ages, the prostate grows and the level of PSA also increases. A high PSA in the blood almost always means that something is wrong with the prostate, but not necessarily that it is prostate cancer. The causes of a high PSA include the benign (non-cancerous) growth that accompanies ageing (benign prostatic hyperplasia, BPH) (see p22), inflammation or infection of the prostate (prostatitis) (see p21) and, least commonly, prostate cancer.

What is the range of PSA levels?

PSA results are returned from the pathology lab expressed as nanograms of PSA per millilitre (ng/mL) of blood. Your PSA test will produce a number and your doctor should try to explain the meaning of that number to you. However this isn't easy because the PSA test is not an accurate test for detecting prostate cancer and understanding what your number means is far from straightforward. It has been conventional to regard a PSA level of 4 ng/ml or higher as "abnormal", and values less than 4 ng/ml as "normal". Results over 4 ng/ml are likely to lead to a recommendation to have a biopsy of the prostate to see why the PSA level is "raised". However, as described above, there are many reasons why PSA levels can rise, without any cancer being present. In fact most men with PSA levels of 4 ng/ml or more don't have prostate cancer. In several studies, about 30% of men with PSA levels of 4 ng/ml or higher were found to have prostate cancer, meaning of course that the other 70% did not have cancer [71].

To complicate things further, having a PSA level less than 4 ng/ml does not mean a man does not have prostate cancer. In one large US study, prostate cancer was diagnosed in 15% of men with PSA less than 4 ng/ml [72]. Because of this, there has been a trend toward dropping the threshold for an "abnormal" PSA test result. In the large European Randomized Study of Screening for Prostate Cancer (more on this study later) the threshold for "abnormal" was dropped from 4 ng/ml to 3 ng/ml. Other experts have suggested different thresholds for "abnormal" according to age, because PSA levels tend to rise with age. According to this approach, a PSA level of up to 2.5 ng/ml is considered normal for a man in his 40s, but a PSA level of up to 6.5 ng/ml is considered normal for a man in his 70s (see Table 8). However there is no evidence to date that these age-adjusted thresholds result in better health outcomes, and there is still no consensus about which threshold(s) should be used to call a result abnormal. For example in 2009, the Urological Society of Australia and New Zealand proposed PSA testing for men from the age of 40 and suggested a PSA level of 0.6 ng/ml be considered "higher risk" for a man aged 40 and a PSA of 0.7 ng/ml be considered "higher risk" for a man aged 50.

Table 8: Upper limits of "normal" for PSA at different age groups (ng/ml)

Age range	Upper limit of normal
40–49	2.5
50–59	3.5
60–69	4.5
70–79	6.5

Source: [73]

While using lower thresholds for an "abnormal" or "higher risk" result has the advantage of detecting more prostate cancers, there are two problems with this approach. The first is that, as we've seen, there is a big reservoir of indolent prostate cancer and there is no evidence that finding all these cancers will be beneficial or result in fewer deaths from prostate cancer. The second is that by dropping the threshold, many more men get caught up in the medical net of "abnormal" or "higher risk" and then have more tests including prostate biopsies. For example, in a community sample of men having PSA tests, using a threshold of 3.5 instead of 4 ng/ml for men aged 50–59 years, twice as many men (4% vs 2%) received an "abnormal" result. Dropping the threshold to 0.7 ng/ml could result in approximately half of all men in this age group receiving a "high risk" result, and being sent for more blood tests and/or biopsies with all the inconvenience, anxiety, risks and costs involved in these extra tests.

In summary, there is no agreement about what constitutes a normal or abnormal PSA level: there is no "threshold" PSA score from which you can conclude that you are or are not highly likely to have prostate cancer. The above studies demonstrate that the PSA test has both poor "sensitivity" (ability to detect cancer if it's there) and poor "specificity" (ability to give a true negative), leading to many false alarms or false positive results. All this means that many men are unnecessarily subjected to prostate biopsies because of the imprecision of the test. And a prostate biopsy is by no means a trivial and risk-free procedure (see p62). Perhaps the only clear thing we can say is that in general, the higher a man's PSA level, the more likely it is that cancer is present.

Dr Richard Ablin, the scientist who discovered the Prostate Specific Antigen in 1970, wrote forcefully about it in March 2010 in *The New York Times*, describing the test's popularity as "a hugely expensive public health disaster". He continued

> the test is hardly more effective than a coin toss. As I've been trying to make clear for many years now, P.S.A. testing can't detect prostate cancer and, more important, it can't distinguish between the two types of prostate cancer — the one that will kill you and the one that won't.

Ablin pulled no punches.

> So why is it still used? Because drug companies continue peddling the tests and advocacy groups push 'prostate cancer awareness' by encouraging men to get screened. Shamefully, the American Urological Association still recommends screening ... Testing should absolutely not be deployed to screen the entire population of men over the age of 50, the outcome pushed by those who stand to profit. I never dreamed that my discovery four decades ago would lead to such a profit-driven public health disaster. The medical community must confront reality and stop the inappropriate use of P.S.A. screening. Doing so would save billions of dollars and rescue millions of men from unnecessary, debilitating treatments. [74]

What happens if you have a high PSA score?

A high PSA score causes concern (and as we have seen, what is meant "high" is by no means clear – it can be in fact as low as 2.5, according to some [73]). But if your doctor interprets your PSA as "high" then two options are available. The first is known as early stage "active surveillance" or "expectant management". Basically, active surveillance at this stage will involve urging you to have more regular PSA tests and probably digital rectal examinations to monitor your prostate.

But the second option is to refer you for a biopsy [75].

What happens when you have biopsy for prostate cancer?

A biopsy involves the extraction of body tissue via a needle so that the tissue can be then examined by a pathologist. The prostate is biopsied through the rectum and the procedure usually takes 10 to 15 minutes. The procedure is performed by a urologist. An ultrasound device is used to view the prostate on a monitor and guide the biopsy needles. A lubricated ultrasound sensor is passed into the rectum. For some this is uncomfortable, but not usually painful.

The biopsy needles are introduced through the shaft of the ultrasound sensor. The needles are then pushed through the rectal wall into the adjacent prostate gland. The needles collect at least 12 samples of prostate tissue which are then sent to a pathologist for testing. A sharp stinging sensation is sometimes experienced. Occasionally the biopsy is not successfully completed and may need to be repeated.

Common side effects of prostate biopsy include:

• pain or discomfort in the rectal area

• distress caused by the sound of the biopsy gun

• anxiety about the biopsy and its results

- blood-stained urine or faeces – this can last up to a week or two. One large Dutch study found blood-stained urine in 23.6% of men [76]
- blood-stained or discoloured semen – this may last for six weeks. The same large study found 45.3% of men had blood in their semen
- difficulty in passing urine – this usually improves quickly.

More serious complications can also arise, although less often. These can include urinary or bowel infection, and far more uncommonly, massive life-threatening rectal bleeding [77], septicaemia (infection of the bloodstream) and even death [78]. In the large Dutch study referred to above, 0.4% (67) of 1687 men who had undergone biopsy had complications serious enough to be admitted to hospital following the procedure. The biopsy needles have to pierce the rectal wall to get to the prostate and bacteria from the bowel may cause an infection. A dose of antibiotic is often given to reduce the risk of infection.

What are the downsides to being told "you have cancer"?

The first consequence of being told that you have cancer in your body is that you henceforth will think of yourself as a man who has cancer. This may seem so obvious as to be hardly worth mentioning, but it bears careful reflection. Knowing that one has cancer can often be an emotionally traumatic experience which can preoccupy some men, causing anxiety and particularly prolonged and repeated periods of depression [6].

But as we have been saying throughout the book, the prostate cancer that you have stands a high chance of being a cancer that may never harm you.

As well, the knowledge that you now have cancer may impact on lives in subtle ways. For example knowing you have prostate cancer may affect your health insurance or life insurance. It can also reverberate around families because it means everyone else now has a relative affected by prostate cancer. That knowledge in turn affects the way doctors and insurance companies will perceive your male relatives as being at higher risk of prostate cancer.

A recent study from Sweden adds important evidence to the debate that getting a prostate cancer diagnosis can increase your risk of having a cardiovascular event or taking your own life. The editors of the highly regarded medical research journal which published the study (*PLoS Medicine*) summarised the study this way:

> The researchers identified nearly 170,000 men diagnosed with prostate cancer between 1961 and 2004 among Swedish men aged 30 years or older by searching the Swedish Cancer Register. They obtained information on subsequent fatal and nonfatal cardiovascular events and suicides from the Causes of Death Register and the Inpatient Register (in Sweden, everyone has a unique national registration number that facilitates searches of different health-related Registers). Before 1987, men with prostate cancer were about 11 times as likely to have a fatal cardiovascular event during the first week after their diagnosis as men without prostate cancer; during the first year after their diagnosis, men with prostate cancer were nearly twice as likely to have a cardiovascular event as men without prostate cancer (a relative risk of 1.9). From 1987, the relative risk of combined fatal and nonfatal cardiovascular events associated with a diagnosis of prostate cancer was 2.8 during the first week and 1.3 during the first year after diagnosis. The relative risk of suicide associated with a diagnosis of prostate cancer was 8.4 during the first week and 2.6 during the first year after diagnosis throughout the study period. [This means that compared with men

not diagnosed with prostate cancer, men given a diagnosis were 8.4 times more likely to commit suicide in the week after being given the news, and 2.6 times more likely in the year after diagnosis.] Finally, men younger than 54 years at diagnosis had higher relative risks of both cardiovascular events and suicide.

These findings suggest that men newly diagnosed with prostate cancer have an increased risk of cardiovascular events and suicide ... these findings strongly suggest that the stress of the diagnosis itself rather than any subsequent treatment has deleterious effects on the health of men receiving a diagnosis of prostate cancer ... this new information should be considered in the ongoing debate about the risks and benefits of PSA screening. [79]

However, another very recent Swedish study which compared men who had had prostate cancer detected after a PSA test with age-matched men without prostate cancer in the general population and also with men with advanced or metastatic prostate cancer found that there was no increased risk of suicide in the newly diagnosed men, whereas the risk was twice as high among men with locally advanced or metastatic disease, compared with the age-matched male population [80].

What do stage, grade and Gleason score mean?

Prostate cancers are often described by their stage, grade, or Gleason score [81].

A cancer's *stage* refers to its extent at diagnosis, in other words, the parts affected by the cancer when it first became evident. Staging is important to both estimating prognosis and selecting treatment. The most common staging system is the TNM system which summarises the extent of the primary tumour (T), spread to local lymph nodes (N), and spread to other parts of the body (M) by assigning numbers to each of these letters.

The most important distinction in staging a prostate cancer is whether or not it appears confined to the prostate. In T1 and T2 cancers, the primary tumour is confined to the prostate, whereas in T3 and T4 cancers, the primary tumour has grown beyond the prostate into adjacent tissues. T1 and T2 cancers are often referred to as "early stage cancers" and have the best outlook, with or without treatment. T3 and T4 are more serious and are often referred to as "locally advanced cancers". N1 cancers have evidence of spread to local lymph nodes, N0 cancers do not. M1 cancers have evidence of spread to other parts of the body, M0 cancers do not. Prostate cancers that have spread to local lymph nodes or beyond are incurable and are referred to as metastatic cancers.

There are several ways of determining evidence of spread beyond the prostate. These include computed tomography (CT or CAT) scans or magnetic resonance imaging (MRI) scans to assess spread within the pelvic region, and radio-isotope bone scans to assess spread into bones. These scans are often called staging tests.

The problem with staging tests is that they are not 100% reliable. The main limitation is that no test is sensitive enough to detect cancer spread at its earliest stages, so a normal result does not rule out the possibility of cancer spread. So while these tests and staging are a helpful guide, they are not conclusive.

Cancers that appear confined to the prostate (T1–2 and N0 and M0) are potentially curable, whereas those that have spread beyond the prostate and its related lymph nodes (M1) are not curable with current treatments. Many prostate cancers involve adjacent tissues (T3–4) or related lymph nodes (N1) at diagnosis; these locally advanced cancers are amenable to treatment, but their curability is controversial.

A cancer's *grade* refers to how aggressive its cells look under a microscope. The *Gleason score* is the standard way of classifying a prostate cancer's grade. It is named after Dr Donald Gleason, a pathologist at the Minneapolis Veterans Affairs Hospital who developed it with other colleagues in the 1960s. The Gleason score reflects how different the tumour looks from normal prostate tissue and suggests how aggressively it is likely to behave.

To calculate the Gleason score for a prostate cancer, the pathologist looks at all available specimens and assigns a score from 1 (least aggressive looking, or low grade) to 5 (most aggressive looking or high grade) to the most common pattern and second most common pattern they see. Adding these numbers together gives the cancer's Gleason score from a minimum of 2 (1+1 = least aggressive, lowest grade) to a maximum of 10 (5+5 = most aggressive, highest grade). In practice, it is unusual for pathologists to report a Gleason score of less than 4 (2+2). Most cancers have Gleason scores between 5 and 10.

A lower Gleason score (5 or less) suggests that the cancer is growing slower, less likely to spread beyond the prostate, and therefore behaving less aggressively. Such cancers are often referred to as "low grade". A higher Gleason score (8 to 10) suggests that the cancer is growing faster, more likely to spread beyond the prostate, and therefore behaving more aggressively. Such cancers are often referred to as "high grade". Most men with prostate cancer have a Gleason score in the middle (6 or 7). These cancers are often referred to as "intermediate grade".

Surviving prostate cancer is more likely with lower Gleason scores (see charts below). This is true with any prostate cancer treatment or watchful waiting. In the charts, "age" means the man's age when the cancer was found. The men in this research study used watchful waiting or hormone treatment. It should also be kept in mind that most men who survived prostate cancer died of other causes.

Tumours with higher Gleason scores (8 to 10) are described as aggressive. They are likely to grow and spread beyond the prostate within five years. Men with higher Gleason score prostate cancers therefore have potentially more to gain from active treatment. However, prostate cancers with higher Gleason scores are also more likely to have spread beyond the prostate and are therefore more difficult to cure.

Age 55 to 59

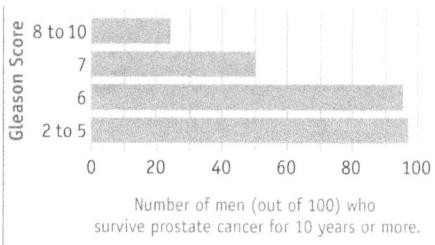

Number of men (out of 100) who survive prostate cancer for 10 years or more.

Age 60 to 64

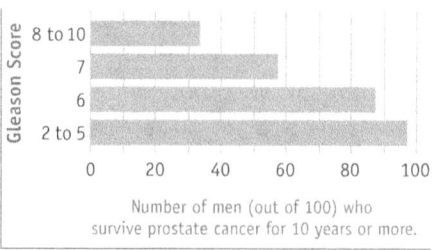

Number of men (out of 100) who survive prostate cancer for 10 years or more.

Age 65 to 69

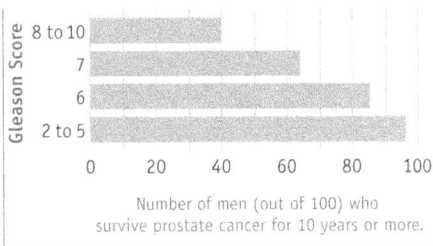

Age 70 to 74

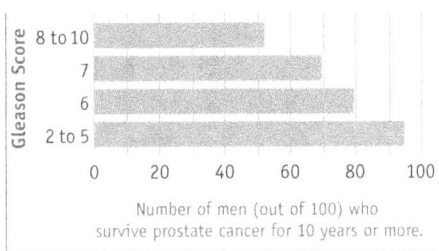

Source: www.effectivehealthcare.ahrq.gov/repFiles/ProstateCancerConsumer.pdf

6

What are the treatments for early stage prostate cancer?

If a prostate biopsy and staging tests reveal an early stage cancer, then a number of options are available to you. The first is active surveillance or "watchful waiting". This is an option frequently offered to men with tumours which have a low Gleason score (e.g. 5 or 6). These cancers are often slow growing, and may never cause you harm. If you opt for watchful waiting, this basically means that for the time being, you and your doctor agree that you will have no treatment but instead, you will undergo regular check-ups (PSA, digital rectal examination, and probably further biopsies). Your doctor will thus know if there is evidence that the cancer is progressing and the risk of spread and further problems is increasing and warrants prostatectomy or radiation.

If you and your doctor decide to treat the cancer, then there are three main options: surgery to remove the cancer; radiation to eradicate the cancer; and hormonal treatment to try to get the cancer under control. Sometimes radiation and hormonal therapy are given in combination. Your doctor may recommend you have hormonal therapy before, during and/or after radiotherapy.

Radical prostatectomy is the complete surgical removal of your prostate. It will only be of potential benefit to men who have early stage prostate cancer which has not spread beyond the prostate. If your cancer has spread (metastasised) beyond the prostate and surrounding tissues, then surgery is unable to eradicate the cancer on its own. A radical prostatectomy is not a minor operation. It is conducted under general anaesthetic. General anaesthetics have their own risks. A radical prostatectomy can be performed "open" through one large incision (5–10 cm), or "laparoscopically", using instruments passed through several smaller incisions.

Retropubic prostatectomy (open) is the most common procedure in Australia. Here, an incision of 8–10 cm is made between the navel and pubic bone through which the prostate and surrounding pelvic lymph nodes are removed. An open retropubic prostatectomy generally takes two and a half to three hours if nerves are not spared and three and a half to four hours if nerves are spared (see below). Removing the prostate means that the part of the urethra travelling through the prostate gland is also removed. The two ends of remaining urethra are then reattached in a connection called an anastomosis.

Perineal prostatectomy is an older open approach, where the prostate is removed through a 5 cm incision in the perineum – the skin and muscles between the scrotum and anus.

Nerve-sparing surgery is designed (as the name implies) to minimise the number of nerves adjacent to the prostate that are damaged during the operation. Bundles of nerves on either side of the prostate are responsible for erections and can be either removed or damaged by surgery. If they remain undamaged, men may have a higher chance of regaining erections after surgery, typically within two to 12 months.

Some may ask why all prostatectomies are not nerve sparing? Surely, good surgeons would always seek to minimise damage to nerves? The problem is that these nerves are small, difficult to identify, fragile, and run along the outer surface of the prostate. Attempts to spare these nerves increase the risk that some prostate cancer will be left behind, particularly if the cancer extends close to where the nerves pass.

Laparoscopic prostatectomy is a newer approach using a thin, tube-like instrument (laparoscope) which allows the surgeon to see inside the abdominal cavity and remove the prostate with other long thin instruments inserted through a series of small incisions. This operation is more demanding for surgeons than open prostatectomy because of the difficulty working through smaller incisions. Recovery times may be quicker because the incisions are smaller, however the operation often takes longer than an open prostatectomy and the risk of cancer recurrence may be higher.

Robotic prostatectomy is an even more recent surgical option that has received a lot of publicity. This involves the urologist using a machine to perform a laparoscopic prostatectomy. The surgeon operates instruments with a console rather than directly. Because it has received so much attention, we deal with this option in greater detail below at page 84.

A highly detailed account of what is involved in radical prostatectomy, including descriptions of problems that can arise can be found on Cornell University's Department of Urology website (www.cornellurology.com/prostate/treatments/prostatectomy.shtml).

Radiotherapy is a potentially curative treatment option when cancer has not spread beyond the prostate. Radiotherapy can also be used to treat symptoms caused by cancer cells that have spread to other parts of the body (metastasised).

External beam radiation therapy (EBRT) is an external radiation therapy used in the treatment of prostate cancer. It is administered by a radiation oncologist after carefully mapping the prostate gland. For early prostate cancer, a typical course of treatment would see you have daily sessions (with weekends off) for four to seven weeks. Each session lasts a few minutes and is painless.

There are two main types of externally delivered radiotherapy: conformal, and IMRT (Intensity-Modulated Radiotherapy). With conformal radiotherapy, the radiotherapy device contours the radiation beams to match the prostate's shape. This seeks to reduce the radiation received by healthy cells in adjacent organs such as the bladder and rectum, therefore reducing the side effects of radiotherapy.

IMRT is a newer, more complex type of conformal radiotherapy and allows the radiotherapist to vary the dose of radiation given to different parts of the tumour and surrounding tissue. It is not yet known whether IMRT is better than conformal radiotherapy.

A perfect session of external beam radiation therapy would affect only the targeted area without causing side effects in surrounding organs. Unfortunately, it is impossible to treat a tumour using external radiation therapy without affecting the surrounding tissues through which the radiation beams must pass.

Brachytherapy (from the Greek *brachy*, meaning "short distance") is radiation therapy delivered directly to a tumour, or from within it, and also known as internal radiotherapy, implant therapy, seed implantation or sealed source radiotherapy. Brachytherapy is commonly used as a treatment for prostate and cervical cancers and can also be used to treat tumours in other parts of the body. Brachytherapy can be used alone or in combination with other therapies such as EBRT and hormonal therapy.

Brachytherapy requires the placement of radiatioactive sources within the tumour under a general or a spinal (epidural) anaesthetic. Around 80–100 small radioactive metal "seeds" can be inserted into the tumour allowing radiation to be released slowly over about six months, after which they are depleted. The seeds are left in the tumour and not surgically removed. They are inserted through the skin between the prostate and the anus, and guided into the prostate gland. Other methods involve the temporary placement of radiatioactive pellets in the tumour for shorter periods over a few days or weeks. As the procedures can cause some swelling of the prostate, which can lead to blockage of the urethra, a catheter is sometimes inserted into the bladder to drain urine. This may be removed after a couple of hours or left in place overnight.

The seeds are not removed and there is little risk of radiation from them affecting other people, although the UK's Macmillan Cancer Support organisation does caution that:

> women who are (or could be) pregnant and children should not stay very close to you for long periods of time. You should not let children sit on your lap, but can hold or cuddle them for a few minutes each day and it is safe for them to be in the same room. [84]

A major advantage of brachytherapy is that the irradiation only affects a very localised area around the radiation seed implants. Exposure to radiation of healthy tissues further away from the sources is therefore reduced. In addition, if the patient moves or if there is any movement of the tumour within the body during treatment, the radiation sources retain their correct position in relation to the tumour. These characteristics of brachytherapy provide advantages over EBRT – the tumour can be treated with very high doses of localised radiation, while reducing the probability of unnecessary damage to surrounding healthy tissues.

A course of brachytherapy can be completed in less time than other radiotherapy techniques. This can help reduce the chance of surviving cancer cells dividing and growing in the intervals between each radiotherapy dose. Patients typically have to make fewer visits to the radiotherapy clinic compared with EBRT, and the treatment is often performed on an outpatient basis. This makes treatment accessible and convenient for many patients.

No randomised trials comparing the efficacy of these various forms of radiotherapy are available.

Hormonal therapy, also known as androgen deprivation therapy (ADT) aims to keep cancer cells from getting the male hormones they need to grow. It is called systemic therapy because it can affect cancer cells throughout the body. Systemic therapy is used to treat cancer that has spread. Sometimes this type of therapy is used to try to prevent the cancer from coming back after surgery or radiation treatment.

There are several forms of ADT. Orchiectomy is a form of surgery to remove the testicles, which are the main source of male hormones. This was introduced in 1942 as the first hormonal treatment for prostate cancer. Although it involves an operation, orchiectomy is considered a hormone therapy because it works by removing the main source of male hormones. Despite sounding drastic, this surgery is simple, quick, and has few risks.

Drugs known as luteinizing hormone-releasing hormone agonists (LHRHA) prevent the testicles from producing testosterone. These drugs are injected or placed as small implants under the skin every one, three or four months. Examples are leuprolide, goserelin and buserelin. All are equally effective. They work by stopping the pituitary gland from releasing hormones that stimulate testosterone production [85].

Drugs known as peripheral anti-androgens block the effects of testosterone in the blood stream on cells in the prostate and elsewhere. These drugs include the "utamides" (bicalutamide, flutamide, nilutamide) and cyproterone. These drugs are usually used to boost the effects of LHRHA or orchidectomy.

So which treatment is best?

There is a shortage of high-level evidence to answer this very obvious and reasonable question. The US Preventive Task Force's 2008 review concluded that "Two recent systematic reviews of the comparative effectiveness and harms of therapies for localized prostate cancer concluded that no single therapy is superior to all others in all situations" [86, 87]. This means that if you decide to be treated for prostate cancer, you and your doctor will need to consider any pre-existing problems that you might have which might be relevant to the treatment you have.

For example, men with urinary problems might be advised against brachytherapy because it can make these symptoms worse. Men with bowel problems would likely be discouraged from external beam radiation therapy because it can affect the rectum as well as the prostate. Nerve-sparing radical prostatectomy is typically selected where high importance is placed on the preservation of sexual function.

Unfortunately, there is no treatment which comes with any assurance or even high probability of avoiding serious unwanted side effects.

Will having a radical prostatectomy save your life?

Let us now assume that you have had a biopsy and staging tests that indicate an "early stage" prostate cancer (T1 or T2, N0, M0). Should you have your prostate removed or should you "watchfully wait" under your doctor's supervision to see if things progress, and then consider medical intervention?

In 2005, *The New England Journal of Medicine* published a study of what happened to 695 men diagnosed with early stage prostate cancer with an average age of 65 years who were randomised to prostatectomy (347 men) or watchful waiting (348 men) [82]. As the men were recruited into the study over several years, the follow-up periods differed, with an average period of eight years. At the time the study reported its results, 83 (23.9%) of the men who had had surgery had died from any cause, compared with 106 (30.5%) of the watchful waiting group. Thirty (8.6%) of the men allocated prostatectomy died from prostate cancer, while 50 (14.4%) of the men allocated to the watchful waiting group died from prostate cancer. We can put this another way: if 1000 similar men with early stage prostate cancer had prostatectomies, then 86 of them will have died from the prostate cancer within the next eight years, while if 1000 similar men were managed with "watchfully waiting" then 144 will have died from prostate cancer. Radical prostatectomy would therefore prevent 58 deaths per 1000 men (an absolute reduction in prostate cancer death of 5.8%, but a 40% reduction if you choose to emphasise the relative risk reduction – see p17).

In 2008, the authors of this study reported results from three more years of follow-up of the men (when the men had been followed for an average of nearly 11 years). By then a total of 137 men in the surgery (radical prostatectomy) group had died compared to 156 of the men in the watchful waiting group. Forty-seven (13.5%) of all the men in the surgery group, compared with 68 (19.5%) of the men in the watchful waiting group had died of prostate cancer [83]. In other words, men who had radical prostatectomy were less likely to die from prostate cancer in the subsequent eleven years than men managed with "watchful waiting." The study also found that men who had radical prostatectomy were less likely to progress to advanced prostate cancer (involving spread of the cancer beyond the prostate gland itself).

What are typical side effects of being treated for prostate cancer?

There is a bewildering range of claims and counterclaims made about adverse side effects of being treated for prostate cancer. When reading websites set up by specialists offering prostate surgery and other treatments, you should note the oblique wording and the use of heavily qualified language ("may", "might", "should", "often", "usually", "commonly") concerning the lack of problems about the treatment that the urologist is offering. Such words are chosen wisely by the owners of such websites because no definite or absolute claims can be made in advance of treatment as the outcome can vary enormously.

Studies looking at the outcomes of medical interventions, including adverse events like serious side effects, should ideally be conducted by researchers who have no competing interests in the results of such studies. For example, a surgeon evaluating his or her own surgical results would always be mindful of the impact of publicity that might follow from results that showed high levels of adverse outcomes. Also patients may be reluctant to complain, or may have little opportunity to complain of side effects to their surgeon, but may feel more able to give an accurate picture of adverse effects to impartial research staff.

This factor is something that all men should keep very much in mind when reading websites or other material that hint that the surgeon being described has a strong success record. It is rare for surgeons to have independently conducted studies evaluating the history of their surgical performance. Many such studies exist but they are almost always without identification so that readers are unable to know to which surgical practice or surgeon they refer. Surgeons are not like musicians or architects whose work can be easily accessed on recordings or by looking at buildings.

When a surgeon advises you on the probabilities of various outcomes occurring, it is always sensible to compare what you are told to the results obtained by independent studies, particularly those which pool together individual studies to provide a synthesis of what a whole range of single studies show when considered together.

The New South Wales study

One very recent study was published by researchers from New South Wales. The researchers approached all men aged less than 70 years living in NSW, who had been diagnosed with histopathologically (laboratory) confirmed prostate cancer, clinical stage T1a to T2c with no evidence of lymph node or distant metastases, between October 2000 and October 2002, and notified to the NSW Central Cancer Registry by May 2003 (or no more than 12 months after their diagnosis). In Australia, all pathology companies, hospitals, radiotherapy centres, day therapy centres, and the registrar of births, deaths and marriages are legally required to notify all cancer cases to the cancer registry in their state. So this is an excellent way of obtaining information about all cases of prostate cancer. It is what we call "population data" as distinct from data obtained from a particular hospital, set of hospitals or individual doctor. The latter are not generally publicly available, and even if such data are available, they may be biased if not all a surgeon's cases are included in the statistics.

In the NSW study, 3195 men were identified as eligible to take part in the study. The 245 doctors treating these men were approached to grant permission for the men to be contacted by the researchers. Eight doctors refused to allow any of their 366 patients to be contacted, and many doctors also declined permission for particular patients to be contacted. Of the 2658 men whose doctors gave permission for contact, 2031 agreed to participate in the study, representing 76.4% of those who were invited.

Table 9: Prevalence of urinary incontinence, bowel problems and sexual impotence, three years after treatment and in untreated controls (percentages). EBRT, external beam radiation therapy; ADT, androgen deprivation therapy.

	Active surveillance ("watchful waiting")	RP total	Nerve sparing RP	Non-nerve sparing RP	EBRT	ADT	Combined EBRT/ADT	Low dose brachy-therapy	High dose brachy-therapy	Controls
Urinary incontinence										
Baseline	6.0	1.1	0.6	1.5	0.0	6.6	3.0	0.0	0.0	1.0
three years	3.4	12.3	9.4	15.1	2.7	4.3	3.9	5.4	7.0	–
Moderate to severe bowel problems										
Baseline	13.5	4.4	3.6	5.3	10.6	10.0	9.0	0.0	2.1	6.3
three years	6.3	3.5	4.1	2.7	14.5	6.4	12.5	0.0	9.3	–
Impotence										
Baseline	27.3	21.5	15.6	27.6	30.2	42.1	39.1	19.0	25.5	22.3
three years	54.3	77.4	67.9	86.7	67.9	97.8	82.3	36.4	72.1	–

Source: [102]

A control group was randomly selected from the electoral roll to enable comparisons with the prevalence of incontinence and impotence problems in men in the community of the same age profile who had not had prostate cancer treatment. The table below summarises the prevalence of sexual and continence problems in the men at follow-up three years later, showing comparisons between the rates experienced by those who had different treatments and the control group, who had had no prostate cancer in that time.

Death

As with many surgical operations, the risk of death from prostate cancer surgery is small but real. The risk is about 0.5% or one in 200 [88, 89]. This risk would be influenced by the older age of many men undergoing surgery. Advanced age is an important independent risk factor for surgical death. A US study of the patient records of 11,522 men who underwent prostatectomy between 1992 and 1996 found that "neither hospital volume nor surgeon volume [i.e. the number of patients the hospital/surgeon has operated on] was significantly associated with surgery-related death" [90]. So if your surgeon ever tries to reassure you about his or her vast experience in performing prostatectomies, or assures you that the hospital where the operation is to be carried out does a high volume of these operations, you should know that the evidence suggests that when it comes to death in the operating theatre as an adverse outcome, these volumes appear to be unrelated to the chance of death being reduced.

Urinary incontinence

The Cochrane Collaboration is an international project designed to synthesise high quality research evidence from all over the world. A Cochrane review allows people to assess the "take-home" messages derived from considering a large number of well-conducted studies, instead of just relying on individual studies, which can differ greatly in what they find. If your surgeon or doctor offers you reassurance about the improbability of incontinence or sexual problems, it would be very wise for you to take note of what the results of all studies *combined* show, and if there is a large difference between what you are told and what the combined research results show, then you would be wise to be circumspect and ask more questions. The Cochrane Library's 2007 updated review of post-prostatectomy urinary incontinence summarised the data on the prevalence of this problem as follows:

> It is not uncommon for men to be incontinent after prostatectomy. The reported frequency varies depending on the type of surgery and surgical technique, the definition and quantification of incontinence, the timing of the evaluation relative to the surgery, and who evaluates the presence or absence of incontinence (physician or patient). Reported prevalence rates of urinary incontinence after radical prostatectomy for prostate cancer vary from 5% to over 60%. For example, in one study at three months after radical prostatectomy, 51% were subjectively wet (self-report) but 36% were wet on pad testing (objective). By 12 months, 20% were subjectively still wet, but only 16% were classed as wet using objective criteria. After transurethral resection for benign prostate disease, urinary incontinence is less common at three months after operation (eg 10% needing to wear pads), but longer term data are not available. After both types of operation, the problem tends to improve with time: it declines and plateaus within one to two years postoperatively. However, some men are left with incontinence that persists for years afterwards. [91]

Table 9 showed that in NSW, compared to the control group, men who had been treated for prostate cancer, regardless of the type of treatment, had higher rates of urinary incontinence three years later. Twelve per cent of men who had had a radical prostatectomy were experiencing urinary incontinence three years later, while rates were lower in those who received various forms of radiation.

According to an August 2008 review by the US Preventive Services Taskforce [92], one year after surgically removing the prostate gland, 15–50% of men have persisting urinary problems. Given that prostate cancer would not have harmed many of these men – i.e., they would have later died from other causes with prostate cancer, but not from it – then this widespread burden of unnecessary surgical side effects is a major downside of the whole push to have men screened [93].

Bowel problems

In the 2009 NSW study which examined men three years after diagnosis and treatment, bowel problems were defined in terms of response to the question, "Overall, how big a problem have your bowel habits been?" with either "moderate" or "big" counting as meaning that the person had a bowel problem. Three years after the treatment, bowel function was consistently worse for all treated men than for men in the control group, but the effect was greatest among men treated with radiation therapy (especially external beam radiation therapy). Table 9 shows that the percentage of men bothered by bowel problems was higher (about double) among men treated with external beam radiation therapy (EBRT) compared to controls.

Sexual impotence

According to the 2008 review by the US Preventive Services Taskforce [92], one year after surgically removing the prostate gland, 20–70% of men have reduced erectile function. As we said above in the case of urinary incontinence, given that prostate cancer would not have harmed many of these men, these widespread side effects of unnecessary surgical treatment are a major weakness of the campaign to have men screened.

Can side effects be reduced if a man is treated by an experienced specialist?

There is evidence that the risk of the side effects (but not risk of death from surgery, see above) of prostatectomy are somewhat lower if the surgery is performed in an institution in which more such operations are performed and by a surgeon who does relatively more operations [90]. The problem here is that consumers are unable to easily find out this information, beyond the assurances that they might be given by their doctor. It is doubtful that many doctors would have access to data on how a given hospital compared to another.

What is the "da Vinci" robotic surgery machine?

The da Vinci robotic surgery machine, used sometimes in prostate cancer surgery, is manufactured by US company, Intuitive Surgical. Like other laparoscopic approaches, it allows a surgeon to perform a prostatectomy through a small incision rather than via the traditional "open surgery" approach. In addition, instead of directly manipulating the instruments, a surgeon using a da Vinci machine sits at a computer console and directs the machine to perform the surgery. The machines cost about $3.5m to buy and $300,000 a year to maintain [94]. Depending on the surgeon and institution involved, robotic surgery prostatectomy can cost in the vicinity of $14,000, which is currently not covered by private health insurance (although the operation could attract the standard Medicare rebate for a radical prostatectomy, which is a small proportion of the cost). In 2006/2007, the average cost for hospital and medical services for a da Vinci prostatectomy was $14,274, of which Medicare pays $2396 (see healthtopics.hcf.com.au/Prostatectomy.aspx).

What is the state of the evidence that robotic surgery is associated with better outcomes for patients? As we will see below, there is currently poor evidence that robotic surgery is demonstrably better.

Even if it *were* true that robotic assisted surgery was demonstrably better for men than regular surgery, these machines are not widely available in Australia, and because of the costs involved, they will be therefore difficult for some men to access or afford. As of 9 August 2010, the da Vinci website shows there to be just eight da Vinci machines in Australia (three in Victoria at Epworth Eastern and Epworth Richmond private hospitals and one at the Peter McCallum Cancer Centre); two in Brisbane (Greenslopes Private Hospital and Royal Brisbane); and one each in Perth (St John of God, Subiaco); Sydney (St Vincent's Private); and Adelaide (Royal Adelaide Hospital). According to a prostate cancer support group website [95], there are just 26 doctors trained in using da Vinci machines in Australia (12 in Melbourne, six in Brisbane, three in Adelaide, three in Sydney and two in Perth).

With the costs involved in the acquisition and maintenance of the machines, there are obvious incentives for those who have invested so heavily in them to promote their use. In May 2006, one Sydney surgeon using the machine made what today can be seen as an astonishingly heroic prediction "I'm convinced that in five years time all prostate operations will be done robotically" [96]. Three years after that prediction, an unknown but certainly a small proportion of men who have had a prostatectomy, have had it done with robotic assistance.

One thing we do know is that the numbers of radical prostatectomies being performed in Australia are rapidly increasing. According to Medicare claims data, the number of radical prostatectomies per year increased approximately fivefold between 1999 and 2009. In 1999, there were 1142 claims for the operation under Medicare

(Item numbers 37210 and 37211) and in 2009 there were 6470. These data are based on services that qualify for a Medicare benefit and for which a claim was processed by Medicare Australia. They do not include services provided by hospital doctors to public patients in public hospital, or services that qualify for a benefit under the Department of Veterans' Affairs National Treatment Account. Medicare statistics are publicly available at www.medicareaustralia. gov.au/statistics/mbs_item.shtml.

Does robotic-assisted surgery produce less adverse outcomes?

The da Vinci corporate website states "studies have shown 'most patients' have a rapid return of sexual function and urinary continence" [97]. "Most" could of course mean as low as 51%. Australian urologists using the machine also allude to better surgical outcomes in their website advertising. Sydney's St Vincent's Hospital's Dr Raji Kooner's website states: "For the patient, da Vinci Prostatectomy may result in more complete eradication of cancer, retention of bladder control and potency" [98]. The Australian Institute for Robotic Surgery website states:

> Robotic-assisted minimally invasive surgery represents an extraordinary technological advance for a broad range of procedures traditionally requiring open surgery. By enabling surgeons to perform complex operations through small incisions, it diminishes the level of patient trauma and helps dramatically improve patient outcomes. [99]

And another: "The potential for an improved and more accurate nerve sparing procedure and preservation of continence". Melbourne's Professor Tony Costello is one of Australia's highest profile prostate surgeons. His personal website (www.tonycostello. com.au/benefits/default.asp?source=cmailer) states that the benefits of robotic surgery "may include reduced risk of incontinence and impotence". But then again, they *may* not.

It is important to note the highly qualified language in these statements ("more complete" [than what?], "may result", "the potential for"). So what is the evidence that robotic assisted surgery produces less adverse outcomes? In October 2009, the prostate cancer debate took yet another interesting turn with a major study published in the *Journal of the American Medical Association* (*JAMA*) [100] throwing a spanner in the works of those who try to play down the extent of adverse outcomes from prostate surgery.

The *JAMA* study of 1938 men followed for five years reported that, compared to routine "retropubic" radical prostatectomy, minimally invasive prostatectomy performed via robotic surgery "was associated with an *increased* risk of genitourinary complications (4.7% versus 2.1%) and diagnoses of incontinence (15.9% versus 12.2%) and erectile dysfunction (26.8 versus 19.2 per 100 person-years)".

In other words, robotic nerve-sparing surgery being promoted by the handful of surgeons who have invested heavily in it actually appears to make things worse. Doctors outlaying such investments plainly have a massive incentive to keep up a healthy throughput of patients using the equipment and one of the ways of doing this is to promote the advantages of better surgical outcomes to their patients.

Dr Phillip Stricker set up the robotic surgery program at Sydney's St Vincent's Hospital. Following the release of the *JAMA* study, in an October 2009 issue of the online medical newsletter *6 Minutes,* he stated that he had performed more robotic prostatectomies than anyone else in NSW, and argued that the *JAMA* results reflected inexperience in the use of the technology, stating that: "it takes time, experience and technique to achieve equal oncological and potency results" and "many of the surgeons who adopt this perform few surgeries and therefore never get off their learning curve".

So what are Australian men to make of such a statement? Dr Stricker seems to be implying that the outcomes in Australia, particularly those obtained by very experienced surgeons like himself, would be different to the results found in the US study.

In fact, Dr Stricker was an author on a very recent paper which compared the results of 502 retropubic radical prostatectomies (RRP) with the results of 212 robot-assisted laproscopic radical prostatectomies (RALP) performed by him between 2006 and the end of 2008 [101]. Stricker and his co-authors reported that when it came to urinary incontinence, it took 200 RALP operations "to achieve equivalent early continence rates to RRP". In other words, it wasn't until Dr Stricker (who had performed more than 2000 RRPs) had performed 200 RALP operations, that the incontinence rates he was achieving were equivalent to those obtained by the RRP approach.

And what about impotency rates? Interestingly, no results were reported. The paper states

> One of the limitations of this study is the short follow-up of 11.2 and 17.2 months for RALP and RRP, respectively. As a result we have not reported any long-term continence outcomes or erectile function in the present study.

With the NSW-wide data showing two thirds of all men undergoing nerve-sparing radical prostatectomy being impotent at three years [102], it is reasonable to assume that one-year rates of impotency will be substantial.

7

To screen or not to screen for prostate cancer?

We now turn to the "crunch" issue in this book, where we will try to provide men with the necessary information to assist them to make a truly informed choice about whether to get tested for prostate cancer.

What is meant by "screening" for a disease?

Screening is a process of identifying asymptomatic people who are at high risk of having or developing a particular disease or condition (often called the "target condition"). Screening has been described as "putting a population through a sieve" (see www.screening.nhs. uk/screening). Most people will pass through the sieve (screening test). These people are called low risk for the target condition; they receive a "normal" test result. Often they are asked to come back in a few years for another test. Some people get caught in the sieve. They are people who are at high (or at least higher) risk of having or developing the target condition. They will be offered follow-up tests to see if they really have the target condition or not. Usually the majority of them do not have the target condition; their experience is described as a "false positive". However, some people really have the target condition (true positives) and they are offered treatment for it. The idea is that this early detection and early treatment of the target condition will produce better results than waiting for the disease or condition to cause symptoms and treating it then.

If it's a good sieve (screening test), it lets through only low-risk people and catches all the high-risk people. Unfortunately none of our sieves are perfect – there are always some people who pass through the sieve who really are high risk and should have been caught (false negatives). Likewise not everyone who gets caught in the sieve actually has the disease or is at high risk of having it. Because our sieves are not perfect, the initial test (the sieve) never definitely tells whether the target condition is present or not. It just sorts people into low risk and high risk for the target condition. So an abnormal screening test always needs to be followed up with more investigations to confirm the initial suspicions.

One of the important things about screening is that the people who are screened (go into the sieve) are *well.* They do not already have the target condition, *or any symptoms of it.* If they do, they are not being screened, they are instead said to be having a "diagnostic" test to see what is the cause of their symptom. For example, a woman with no symptoms of breast cancer (such as a breast lump) may be screened by a mammogram. If her screening mammogram is abnormal, she will then be offered follow-up tests (which may include more mammograms, an ultrasound and/or a biopsy) to establish whether she has breast cancer or not. These follow-up tests may be called diagnostic tests, because they are done to establish a diagnosis, after the initial screening test has indicated she has something suspicious. A woman who already has a breast lump will also have a *diagnostic* mammogram to see if the lump is cancer or not. Even though it is the same test (a mammogram) this is not screening, this is diagnosis because she already has something suspicious (a lump). Her mammogram does not lead to the possibility of treating the cancer early, before it has caused any symptoms.

Another very important point about screening is that the screening test alone does not deliver any benefit. It is the package of the screening test *plus early treatment* that may deliver a health benefit.

Just doing the test is only the first step of a screening program. Without an effective program which provides the follow-up test(s) and early, effective treatment for people who have the target condition, screening cannot possibly do any good. So it is best to think of screening as a screening *program*, rather than a screening *test*.

In Australia, blood taken from a heel prick of newborn babies is routinely screened to help identify over 20 metabolic conditions such as phenylketonuria (PKU – an enzyme deficiency disorder which if left untreated, can lead to mental retardation); homocystinuria (an inherited enzyme deficiency disease involving a build-up of the amino acid homocystine which can cause progressive mental retardation) and maple syrup urine disease (named after the presence of sweet-smelling urine in affected babies. If left untreated, infants suffer severe brain damage and eventually die.)

Screening of adults seeks to find evidence of chronic disease not yet causing symptoms and therefore not under medical care and may identify risk factors like high cholesterol and blood pressure, genetic pre-disposition or early evidence of disease – as is the case with colorectal, cervical and breast cancer screening.

Why do we screen for some diseases but not others?

In 1968, the World Health Organization published what would become a classic report in the history of modern medicine [103]. It set out a framework for deciding when it is worthwhile to screen. While it set out some very useful principles, it has been updated several times since as we have learnt more about screening and its pitfalls. For example in 2003, the National Screening Unit in New Zealand published a short set of criteria (see Table 10). Similar criteria have been developed and adopted to guide policy in the UK, Canada and the US.

Table 10: Criteria for assessing screening programs

The condition is a suitable candidate for screening.

There is a suitable test.

There is an effective and accessible treatment or intervention for the condition identified through early detection.

There is high quality evidence, ideally from randomized controlled trials, that a screening program is effective in reducing mortality and morbidity.

The potential benefit from the screening programme should outweigh the potential physical and psychological harm (caused by the test, diagnostic procedures and treatment).

The health care system will be capable of supporting all necessary elements of the screening pathway, including diagnosis, follow-up and program evaluation.

There is consideration of social and ethical issues.

There is consideration of cost-benefit issues.

Source: www.nsu.govt.nz/files/NSU/Screening_to_improve_health.pdf

These criteria are very important. Although it seems odd, a screening program which does not address these criteria may in fact do more harm than good. This is because screening is done to well people, so there is a real possibility of doing harm if the screening test or the following tests or the treatment for the target condition carry important risks. For this reason there is now broad agreement among expert groups that there must be "gold standard" evidence (mostly this means evidence from randomised controlled trials) that detecting disease early and treating it earlier than would otherwise have happened must reduce deaths or improve quality of life. In short, if treating a person's disease at a very early time makes no positive difference to their life, why would you do it? You would be running the risk of giving people only more "disease-time" rather than more lifetime. The idea of adverse effects (or harmful effects) of screening is quite counterintuitive. But it is reasonable to think that all screening will do some harm.

Sometimes the harm is limited to the anxiety and inconvenience of undergoing the screening test. However it is vital to appreciate that screening is actually a "package deal" of early detection *and* early treatment if disease or pre-disease is found. If you don't go on to treat what you find, there can be no benefit of screening. For example, what is the point of finding out your child has PKU if you are not going to do anything to modify their diet? Similarly is there really any point in finding out early you have breast or bowel cancer if you don't intend to treat it? Therefore the adverse effects of treating screen-detected disease have to be considered as adverse effects of screening. And that's very important in prostate cancer screening because as we saw earlier, adverse effects of follow-up tests and treatments for prostate cancer are common and can be severe.

The side effects of prostate cancer treatment are especially relevant when thinking about the "package deal" of prostate cancer screening because of the big reservoir of indolent (non-harmful) prostate cancer that we talked about before. This big reservoir of indolent prostate cancer in the population means that if we screen whole populations of men for the disease, we will find it in many of them. If we treat all those people, there is enormous potential to cause harmful effects in many men. This means it's especially important in the case of prostate cancer screening to carefully consider whether the benefits of screening are likely to outweigh the harms. Soon we will take a detailed look at what we really know about the benefit of prostate cancer screening.

Health agencies around the world are increasingly recognising that many people want to be involved in decisions that affect their own health. Many people no longer want their doctor or their government to decide for them. Especially in "close-call" decisions where the beneficial effects and harmful effects may be finely balanced and in decisions where personal preferences may strongly influence what a person wishes to do, people want to have a say. Screening for prostate cancer is perhaps the best example available of such a "close call" and of what people studying this phenomenon call a "preference-sensitive decision" [104]. The US Preventive Services Taskforce assessment of the evidence for and against PSA screening concluded: "the current evidence is insufficient to assess the balance of benefits and harms of prostate cancer screening in men younger than 75 years". In short, it is a close call; there are potential benefits and harms, and whether you think the benefit is worth the risk is a matter of personal judgement. This is why the Taskforce, and other health agencies such as Cancer Council Australia, Andrology Australia, the UK National Screening Committee and the National Screening Unit in NZ all suggest that men should be adequately informed about the pros and cons of PSA screening before going ahead with a PSA screening test.

What is the benefit of screening for prostate cancer?

Let's now take a careful look at what we really know about whether screening for prostate cancer saves men from dying early from prostate cancer. We will look at a "randomised clinical trial" or a "randomised controlled trial" in relation to prostate cancer screening to see how do these trials differ from other "studies" about the effectiveness of screening.

In short, "randomised clinical trials" or "randomised controlled trials" provide a much higher level of evidence than other "observational studies".

Many research reports published in the medical literature are what are known as "observational studies". An example of a basic observational study would be when a group of people who smoke are followed for a long time, maybe 20 years, to see how many people develop lung cancer, heart disease and so on. Their results are compared with a control group of non-smokers who are also followed for the same time. The temptation is to see any differences in the disease patterns of the two groups as being attributable to (here) the smoking and nothing else. While these studies are sometimes very important they have a big weakness, which is that you can never be sure that the exposed group (in this example the smokers) aren't different in some important way from the control group (in this example the non-smokers). For example, the non-smokers may be healthier in other ways such as exercising more or eating better, and it could be these differences that are important rather than the smoking itself (although with this example, the weight of evidence is overwhelming that smoking is so risky that it overwhelms all other considerations).

We now have many examples of how we have been misled by relying on these kinds of observational studies. A recent example was hormone therapy (HT) and heart disease. On the basis of observational studies, it was long believed that HT should lower the risk of heart disease in post-menopausal women and on this basis many women around the world were prescribed HT for many years for this and other possible benefits. However when the big randomised controlled trials were finally done, it was clear that HT does not prevent heart disease in these women and may even increase the risk. In short, we learnt the hard way that relying on observational studies to decide what works in health care isn't good enough. And this is particularly true of screening when it's very easy to be misled by observational studies as there can be many, and subtle, differences between screened and non-screened people.

So instead we rely on randomised controlled trials (RCTs) in prostate cancer screening. These provide much stronger evidence because we compare two groups of people – men who have been allocated at random (in a process like a lottery) to be screened with men who have been allocated at random to no screening. This means there shouldn't be any important differences between the groups we are comparing other than participation in prostate cancer screening.

With an RCT examining the power of PSA testing to save lives, men in the at-risk age group (over 50) who have not had a PSA test are randomly allocated either to the "intervention" group (i.e. they will be asked to have a PSA test every year or few years) or to the "control" group (i.e. they are not given a PSA test). The men in both groups are then followed by researchers over a number of years to see what happens to them. Here, the main outcomes of interest are simply "what proportion of men in the intervention and control groups develop prostate cancer, and what proportion die from it?"

When it comes to RCTs examining the impact of PSA screening on death from prostate cancer, the first challenge is to find large populations of men who have not already had a PSA test. In the USA, the promotion and uptake of PSA screening has been so large that a recent long-awaited RCT examining whether prostate screening saves lives was badly affected by many of those who were assigned to the "no screening group" in fact getting screened. "Rates of screening in the control group increased from 40% in the first year to 52% in the sixth year for PSA testing and ranged from 41 to 46% for digital rectal examination" [105]. This "corruption" of the control group badly affected the ability of the study to test whether screening made any difference in preventing death. The published results of the US trial showed no survival benefit from screening but because of this trial "corruption", that study provides little insight into whether screening "works".

Does screening for prostate cancer save lives?

Our knowledge of this advanced significantly in 2009 with the publication of a major nine-year-long study, the European Randomized Study of Screening for Prostate Cancer (ERSPC) [18]. In this large RCT study, the prostate cancer death rate in men who were screened was compared with the rate in men who were not screened. If early detection were beneficial, we would expect that in the screened group, that there would be a lower rate of death from prostate cancer because many life-threatening cancers would have been detected early and the men put through treatment. If it were true that early detection and treatment of men saved lives, the rate of death from prostate cancer in the screened men should be lower than in the non-screened men.

The ERSPC [18] commenced in the early 1990s. The study included 182,000 men aged 50 to 74 years from seven European countries. Some of these men were randomly assigned to a group that was offered PSA screening at an average of once every four years (average 2.1 tests in the nine years). Others were assigned to a control group that did not receive such PSA testing. The primary outcome of interest to the study authors was the rate of death from prostate cancer.

During a median follow-up of nine years, the cumulative incidence of prostate cancer diagnosed in the screened men was 82 per 1000 men and 48 per 1000 men in the control group. Basically this means that in the nine years after the men were first screened, nearly double the rate of prostate cancers was found in men who were screened at an average of once every four years than was found in the men who were not offered screening. The prostate cancers found in the non-screened control group would have been found because some of these men would have experienced symptoms and gone to see a doctor. Investigations would have then found prostate cancer in these men.

So far then, we can say that by screening lots of men, we will find nearly twice as many histologically (laboratory) confirmed cancers in those screened men than in men who don't get screened but who present to doctors with symptoms which are then investigated and found to be cancer. But what we really need to know is how many men in the screened and unscreened groups died from prostate cancer in the nine years of the study, the main focus of interest.

The results were 2.94 deaths per 1000 men in nine years in the group of screened men. In the control group, there were 3.65 deaths per 1000 men in nine years. The difference means that screening prevented just 0.71 deaths per 1000 men over nine years. This is about a 20% reduction (in relative terms) in the risk of dying from prostate cancer (0.71/3.65). Now that might not sound very much, but nine years isn't very long in the course of a slow disease like prostate cancer. Also as we can readily see, dying from prostate cancer is uncommon in men this age, so as we expect, the death rate is low in both groups. In other words it is hard to see a big effect because the outcome is relatively uncommon to start with.

This compares well with the results of randomized studies of mammographic screening for breast cancer in women. Systematic reviews of these trials conclude that among women aged 50–69 years screening with mammograms produces a relative benefit of about 15% [106].

The key issue that all men need to consider, however, is the balancing of benefits versus harms. So the ERSPC study found that we can reduce the risk of dying from prostate cancer from 3.65 deaths per 1000 men over nine years to 2.94 deaths per 1000 men over nine years. The price of this modest benefit is the extra numbers of men diagnosed with and treated for prostate cancer. Instead of having 48 per 1000 men affected by a prostate cancer diagnosis and treatment, as in the control group, there were 82 men affected in the screened group, in order to prevent less than one death per 1000 men. Whether you think that is a reasonable price to pay depends on how you feel about the psychological and physical side effects of having a prostate cancer diagnosis and treatment (more on that below).

The investigators of the study used these numbers to calculate that 1410 men would need to be screened and 48 additional cases of prostate cancer would need to be treated to prevent a single death from prostate cancer. For some readers, this might be a bit hard to follow. Put another way, suppose these 48 men were to gather in one room. Each of them would be convinced that the detection and treatment of their prostate cancer had saved their life. And 47 of the 48 would be wrong.

The following may also help. *The New York Times* ran a report on PSA screening on 19 March 2009 [107] describing the study as "the first based on rigorous randomized trials". In summarising the results, the *NYT* quoted Dr Peter Bach, a physician and epidemiologist at Memorial Sloan-Kettering Cancer Center. Bach suggested that one way to think of the results of the European trial was to consider a man having a PSA test that needed further investigation:

> It leads to a biopsy that reveals he has prostate cancer and he is treated for it. There is a one in 50 chance that in 2019 or later he will be spared death from a cancer that would otherwise have killed him. And there is a 49 in 50 chance that he will have been treated unnecessarily for a cancer that was never a threat to his life.

Before we leave this study, some other results from it were that in the screening group, 82% of men accepted at least one offer of screening. During the trial, 126,462 PSA-based tests were performed on men in the screening group. In total, 16.2% of these tests were positive and 85.8% of the men with positive PSA results took up the recommendation to have a biopsy. Of the men who underwent biopsy, 75.9% had a false positive result (in other words, their elevated PSA did not translate to laboratory confirmed prostate cancer). The proportions of men who had a Gleason score of 6 or less were 72.2% in the screening group and 54.8% in the control group, and the proportions with a Gleason score of 7 or more were 27.8% in the screening group and 45.2% in the control group. This is to be expected because screening detects cancers earlier, and also, as we have seen, finds many low grade cancers.

While we have tried to explain the complexities of the European trial carefully to maximise its comprehensiveness to men without epidemiological training, we appreciate that for some its meaning will still be unclear. Over the next pages we present the "take-home" messages in graphic form via diagrams with a single dot representing one of a 1000 men. We hope this information will assist in your understanding.

Source: Data from the European Randomized Study of Screening for Prostate Cancer; illustrations by Erin Mathieu, Sydney School of Public Health, University of Sydney

1000 men aged 55-69 who DO NOT have PSA screening

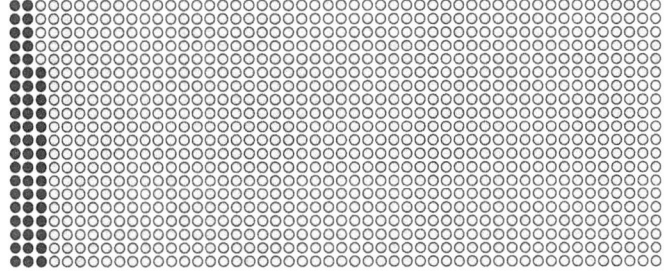

55 men will have prostate cancer
detected over 10 years

1000 men aged 55-69 who have PSA screening

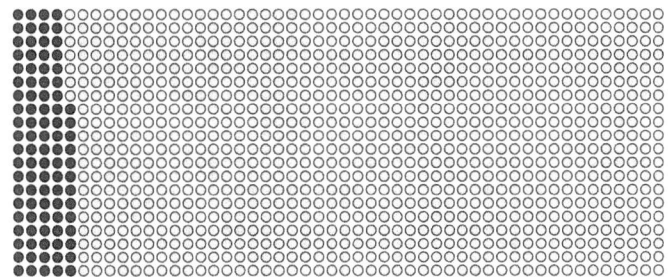

93 men will have prostate cancer
detected over 10 years

1000 men aged 55-69 who DO NOT have PSA screening

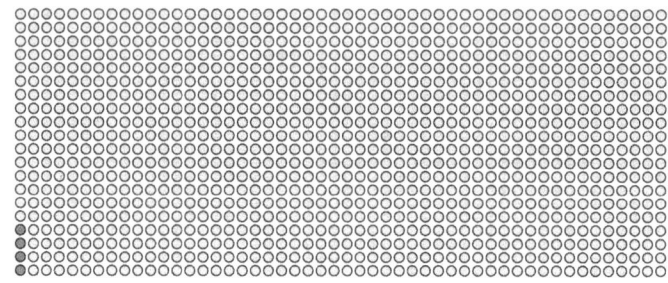

4 men will die from prostate cancer
over 10 years

1000 men aged 55-69 who have PSA screening

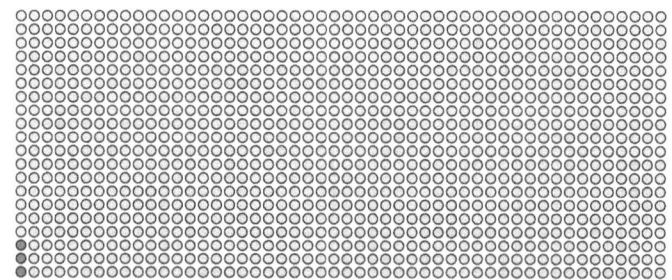

3 men will die from prostate cancer
over 10 years

The 2010 Swedish Göteborg study

The Göteborg (Sweden) trial was a randomised controlled trial in which men aged 50–64 were randomly allocated to no screening or PSA screening every two years. After 14 years of follow-up, the study found that PSA screening reduced the men's chances of dying of prostate cancer by nearly half. Over 14 years, 0.5% of the men in the screened group (that is 0.5 per 100 men, or one man in every 200 men) died from prostate cancer compared with 0.9% of the men in the control group who were not screened (0.9 per 100 men or just under one in every 100 men). Being screened also (unsurprisingly) increased the men's chances of having prostate cancer diagnosed; over 14 years, 12.7% of the men in the screened group were diagnosed with prostate cancer compared with 8.2% of the men in the control group. Treatments for screening detected cancers included radical prostatectomy (about 40%), radiation therapy (8%), hormone therapy (7%), surveillance followed by treatment (15%) and surveillance only (about 30%).

Expressed another way, the results of this study were that compared to a situation of no screening, 293 men need to be invited for PSA screening and 12 additional men will be diagnosed with (and treated for) prostate cancer to prevent one death from prostate cancer over 14 years.

These results are considerably better than those obtained in the European multi-nation trial. So which study is more important in the Australian debate? Which "take-home" message is most important for Australian men to consider? A commentary [33] published in *Lancet Oncology* in the same issue as the trial results sought to answer the question "why are there these differences between ERSPC and Göteborg?" The University of Cambridge's David Neal addressed this important question this way:

Probably the most important points are the longer length of time since randomisation and the younger age at screening than in the ERSPC, in a national context of a low baseline rate of PSA testing before the study ... The [Göteborg] study by Hugosson and colleagues might be generalisable to populations that have not had prior extensive PSA testing, but probably not generalisable to populations that have had such testing – eg, in the Göteborg study only 56% of cancers were low-risk according to the D'Amico criteria, by contrast with tumours found in the second or additional rounds of screening in the ERSPC, and particularly with tumours found in the course of PSA testing in the USA, where typically low-risk cancers would be found in 75% of patients.

This point was also made in a commentary published by the US National Cancer Institute:

During the course of the trial, the state of prostate cancer screening in Sweden was "very different from the situation in the United States right now," explained Dr. Eric Klein, chair of the Glickman Urological and Kidney Institute at the Cleveland Clinic. "It's comparable to when PSA was introduced in the United States in the late '80s. Now we have a heavily screened population, which is why it makes sense to build on the results of this trial to further refine our screening efforts to identify men at risk for potentially lethal cancers." (see www.cancer.gov/ncicancerbulletin/071310/page5)

Like the USA, Australia is a nation which has had extensive "de facto" screening of the population for at least 10 years with more than 50% of men having been tested at least once [16]. This means that the Australian population, many of whom have already been tested, might be expected to show less benefit of screening than was found in Goteborg.

What are the harmful effects of screening for prostate cancer?

Overdiagnosis: cancer treatments you didn't need

As we have emphasised throughout the book, there is a big risk with PSA testing of dredging up cancers that would have remained silent and not caused symptoms throughout life. These cancers would only be found if the person happened to have an autopsy after they died (or if they were screened for prostate cancer).

These cancers are called overdiagnosed cancers. Unfortunately our tests are not yet good enough to distinguish between overdiagnosed cancers and symptom-causing, life-threatening cancers. So we offer treatment to everyone with prostate cancer. These cancer treatments commonly have adverse effects and sometimes those adverse effects can be really bad for a person's quality of life; they can be long lasting or even life threatening. This makes overdiagnosis and consequent overtreatment the number one harmful effect of prostate cancer screening.

The US Preventive Health Task Force's 2008 review of the evidence [13] on prostate screening concluded that

> Modeling studies based on U.S. incidence data suggest over-diagnosis rates ranging from 29% to 44% of all prostate cancer cases detected by PSA screening [108]. Because patients with 'pseudo-disease' receive no benefit from, and may be harmed by, prostate cancer screening and treatment, prostate cancer detection in this population constitutes an important burden.

Thanks to the results from the ERSPC nine-year trial of screening [18], we know that about one in 48 men with screen-detected prostate cancer will have death from prostate cancer prevented by screening (see above). This means the other 47 men have prostate cancer which is overdiagnosed and overtreated, in the sense that it would not have killed them had it not been found and not treated. Recall however, that the follow-up time of the European trial was only nine years. It is possible that had the trial gone for longer (say 20 or 30 years) more of these 48 men may have benefited and had a prostate cancer death averted. This seems very plausible because as we saw earlier, prostate cancer deaths increase with age. On the other hand it's possible the number of prostate cancer deaths prevented might not have got any greater had the trial gone for longer. We just don't know.

As we saw, the Göteborg study published data on the number of men who could be expected to benefit from screening, that is, prevent death from prostate cancer. They estimated that about one in 12 men with screen-detected prostate cancer will have death from prostate cancer prevented by screening within a time frame of 14 years. This means only 11 men would have been overdiagnosed and overtreated prostate cancer. This better result is likely due to a combination of factors including the longer length of follow-up time (14 years rather than nine years) and the difference in study population (that is men who were largely unscreened for prostate cancer). It is likely that the numbers for Australian men would lie somewhere between these two estimates.

What we do know is that, regardless of which study you elect to put your faith in, the vast majority of men who have prostate cancer found by PSA testing do not benefit, or in other words, do not have a prostate cancer death prevented. It's also pretty clear that if you have screening-detected prostate cancer found and treated you are much, much more likely to be experiencing overdiagnosis and overtreatment than you are to be having a prostate cancer death prevented.

False alarms

While overdiagnosis may be the biggest downside of PSA screening, false alarms are a considerable problem too. In the European study, 16% of PSA tests were abnormal leading men to have a biopsy. About a quarter of these men were found to have prostate cancer on their follow-up biopsy. In other words, about 75% (three quarters) of men who had a biopsy triggered by a raised PSA test result experienced a false alarm [18]. This means they had an abnormal PSA test result but their subsequent prostate biopsy showed no cancer. There are both psychological and physical downsides of having a false alarm. Some people describe it as the scariest time of their lives. For most, it is at least inconvenient, uncomfortable and anxiety provoking to some extent [109]. While most people (more than 90%) do not experience any important physical adverse effects of the biopsy, a few people (less than 1%) suffer important complications particularly infection, which can be serious enough to require intravenous antibiotics and hospitalisation [87].

It is important to remember that the chance of experiencing a false alarm increases as you have more screening tests. So while the chance of having a false alarm is in the range 3–10% following one PSA test, if you have tests on a regular basis (say yearly or every two years) the chance of having a false alarm after one of them becomes quite high over a "lifetime" of screening.

Make your own choice: weighing up the benefits and harmful effects of prostate cancer

As mentioned earlier, there is considerable interest in providing men with decision tools to help them weigh up the benefit versus risks of PSA screening. A number of these "decision aids" have been developed and tested in the US, Canada and the UK. One such decision aid, Prosdex, was developed and evaluated in Wales. It is available for free online at www.prosdex.com

8

Some further questions and answers

What is the difference between "screening" and "testing" for prostate cancer?

A s explained, "screening" means that people with no signs or symptoms of disease are urged to undergo a test to see if they have that disease. Because (except in rare circumstances) people cannot be compelled to be screened, governments sometimes mount large-scale public awareness campaigns designed to inform and persuade those people for whom screening is relevant to go to either a special screening service or to see their doctor (if the screening can be done in a doctor's rooms). Essentially then, screening is testing people on a mass scale who have no symptoms of disease to see if indicators of disease may be present.

Those who try to distinguish "testing" from "screening" are in effect playing semantic games. Those urging that men be tested seldom use the term "screening", but by directing the message at all men aged over 50, their intention is to effectively promote wholesale screening. They are in fact promoting screening but calling it "testing". They are often aware of the long list of expert bodies (see p7) which have examined the wisdom of promoting screening and concluded that it is not a policy that should be promoted. But these groups are seeking to have it both ways by rejecting "screening" but supporting mass testing – in effect the same thing. A good example of this is the current policy of the Urological Society of Australia and New Zealand. Their policy states:

1. Prostate cancer is a major health problem and is the second leading cause of male cancer deaths in Australia and New Zealand. The Urological Society of Australia and New Zealand (USANZ) currently **does not recommend the use of mass population-based Prostate Specific Antigen (PSA) screening** as public health policy, as published studies to date have not taken into account the cost effectiveness of screening, nor the full extent of over-detection and over-treatment.

2. However, based on recent data from one of two large randomised screening studies, there was a reduced risk of prostate cancer death with PSA testing and treatment in those patients in the 55–69 year age group after 7–8 years. Therefore **PSA based testing, together with digital rectal examination (DRE), should be offered to men in this age group**, after providing information about the risks and benefits of such testing. [110] [our emphasis]

This policy is plainly having a bet each way. It agrees that screening all men is not a good idea for the reasons we explain in detail in this book (overdetection and overtreatment) but in the very next paragraph, states that PSA "testing" should be "offered" to men after age 55. This is simply a "Clayton's" screening policy: promoting screening when you are not promoting it.

If women are screened for breast cancer, shouldn't men be screened for "their" cancer too?

Women have their cancer screening tests (for cervical and breast cancer) and the Australian government recommends that all people aged over 50 be screened regularly for colorectal (bowel) cancer, so doesn't it makes sense that men should be screened for prostate cancer?

In media coverage of the disease, men are repeatedly told they are not "being a man" if they don't get tested. This is an argument frequently advanced by prostate screening advocates. Its subtext is that women are somehow more sensible about their health than men because more of them are attuned to regularly doing the sensible thing and checking for cancer. The simplistic logic runs that men should behave like women and line up to be tested too. This argument ignores any consideration of all the evidence that we have summarised, and ignores the rather important difference that the best available evidence shows a modest benefit of screening which must be weighed against the substantial risk of harm through overdiagnosis and overtreatment.

The parallel with mammography screening is an interesting one. Both PSA screening and mammography screening are double-edged swords. Both have a benefit (reduced chance of dying from cancer) and both have adverse effects which range from mild to severe. Like PSA screening we have evidence from randomised trials that mammography screening reduces women's chances of dying from breast cancer. The effect is a little different, however, because breast cancer is a more common cause of death among women in their 40s, 50s and 60s than prostate cancer is among men in these age groups (as we have seen, most prostate cancer deaths occur in men aged over 70, and the average age of death from prostate cancer is almost 80). So compared to PSA screening, more relatively young women benefit from mammography screening.

Breast cancer screening has downsides too, just as we have seen with prostate cancer screening. A woman who has mammography screening may experience a false alarm by receiving an abnormal result on her mammogram which turns out not to be breast cancer, just like a man may get a high PSA level which turns out not to be prostate cancer. It may take several tests, often involving a biopsy, to confirm she does not have breast cancer. This can be very anxiety provoking.

More importantly, overdiagnosis and overtreatment are also problems with mammography screening. Strange though it may seem, a woman may be diagnosed with screen-detected breast cancer which is indolent and never destined to become life threatening. In fact it is estimated that about 25–30% of breast cancers found by screening may be like this [111, 112]. Because we can't distinguish aggressive, life-threatening breast cancer from indolent breast cancer, all women diagnosed with breast cancer are offered treatment. In this way, the overdiagnosis becomes overtreatment. And as with prostate cancer, a diagnosis of breast cancer can have profound psychological effects, and treatments for breast cancer may have serious adverse physical effects.

With PSA screening, 12–50 extra men may be diagnosed with prostate cancer for each man whose death from prostate cancer is averted by screening. With mammography screening there is also a wide range of estimates about how many extra women are diagnosed with and treated for breast cancer. Some researchers estimate that two extra women are diagnosed with breast cancer for each woman whose death from breast cancer is averted by mammography screening. Others estimate 10 extra women are diagnosed with breast cancer for each woman whose death from breast cancer is averted [113]. This means, the balanace of benefits to harms of screening for breast cancer is better, as fewer extra women are treated to prevent each death from breast cancer.

Is improved treatment for prostate cancer responsible for decreasing death rates from prostate cancer?

As we demonstrated earlier, death rates from prostate cancer are now at about the same level that they were in the 1970s. In 1968 the age-adjusted death rate for prostate cancer was 35.6 per 100,000 and in 2007 it was 31 per 100,000 (see Table 4). This small difference follows the massive population-wide numbers of men who have been tested, investigated and treated for prostate cancer in this 39-year period. While it is possible that both improved treatment and screening with the PSA test are contributing to the decline in death rates observed since the early 1990s (i.e. from a high of 43.7 per 100,000 in 1993 to 31 per 100,000 in 2007), it seems clear that neither is having a very impressive impact.

Do male doctors and cancer experts themselves get tested for prostate cancer?

We know that smoking rates among doctors are the lowest in the population: in 1996, just 2% of Australian doctors admitted to smoking [114]. So do Australia's male doctors aged over 50 also "take their own medicine" when it comes to being tested for prostate cancer? One 2002 study from Victoria has given us information on this. It found a minority – 45% – of doctors aged 49 or more had been tested [115]. By contrast, a 2006 US study found much higher levels of testing (95% of urologists and 78% of non-urologists) [116].

Who benefits from mass PSA testing in Australia?

One reason why so many men are now asking to be tested lies in the promotional activities of powerful commercial forces which strategically promote the benefits of testing but rarely talk about the major downsides. The US-based Us Too! International with

325 worldwide groups is promoted as a "grassroots" organisation established and run by prostate cancer survivors wanting to assist men with making an "informed" choice. The Us Too! website lists a formidably long list of corporate sponsors in the pharmaceutical, medical equipment and pathology service industries [117]. All of these industries of course stand to benefit financially by large numbers of men being tested and investigated. It is thus predictable that the organisation recommends annual PSA tests for men, despite the controversies described in this book [118].

The strategy of drug and biotech companies supporting and funding apparently spontaneously created grassroots community groups of people living with a disease is known as "astroturfing". Wikipedia describes astroturfing like this:

> Astroturfing [refers to] political, advertising, or public relations campaigns seeking to create the impression of being spontaneous "grassroots" behaviour, hence the reference to the artificial grass, AstroTurf. The goal of such a campaign is to disguise the efforts of a political or commercial entity as an independent public reaction to some political entity – a politician, political group, product, service, or event. Astroturfers attempt to orchestrate the actions of apparently diverse and geographically distributed individuals, by both overt ("outreach", "awareness", etc.) and covert (disinformation) means. Astroturfing may be undertaken by an individual pushing a personal agenda or highly organized professional groups with financial backing from large corporations, non-profits, or activist organizations. Very often the efforts are conducted by political consultants who also specialize in opposition research.

So when you hear about an organisation promoting prostate cancer screening, it is a good idea to try and investigate whether the organisation is sponsored by those who will benefit by large numbers of men getting tested.

In Australia, the Prostate Cancer Foundation's website lists a large number of commercial sponsors of the Foundation. Among these are four pharmaceutical companies and the da Vinci company, which makes the robotic surgical machine discussed earlier. Each of the four pharmaceutical companies sells diagnostics (PSA tests) or drugs used to treat prostate cancer. That sounds like a natural and obvious coincidence of interests. The Foundation is dedicated to fighting prostate cancer and the companies have products that are involved in that fight. Well and good. But you will look in vain on the Foundation's website or in any of its literature for any detailed explanation of the other side of the debate about prostate cancer screening that might cause some men to take pause.

To sum up

Prostate cancer is the second greatest cause of cancer death in Australian men after lung cancer. Like most cancers, it is a disease which is very uncommon to rare in men aged less than 50, although it does of course kill some men in their 40s and 50s. This alone will be news to many men who have heard about prostate cancer in the news and heard people saying that it can kill men young.

In fact, prostate cancer is a disease which – more than any other cancer – tends to kill men very late in life in the years in which men are at higher risk from dying per se (i.e. from any cause). Prostate cancer is one of the diseases that brings down the final curtain late in life in men. We all will die from some disease.

In 2010, the Prostate Cancer Foundation of Australia ran television ads featuring Australian male celebrities urging all men over 50 and men over 40 with a family history of the disease to get tested. The line-up included cricketers and footballers in their 30s. *Underbelly* actor Daniel Amalm, 31, was one of several young men who said on camera that prostate cancer can kill men "just like me". But of the 75,433 men who died from prostate cancer between 1968 and 2007 in Australia, just two (0.003%) were aged 30–34. Given that no government anywhere in the world, no peak cancer control agency, and no high level, independent review of the evidence has to date supported screening, it is important to question campaigns like the Foundation's and consider what it might achieve if it was wildly successful.

Prostate cancer screening advocates repeatedly emphasise that men need to make informed decisions about being tested. We wrote this book to provide men with information that is rarely included in "pro-screening" public information about prostate cancer.

Some incontestable information that you won't find on the Prostate Cancer Foundation's website nor in its TV ads is as follows.

First, prostate cancer is a disease that far more men die *with* rather than *from*. As we saw, we know this thanks to many autopsy studies where men who die suddenly or without having recently seen a doctor are examined for cause of death. At autopsy, 10–20% of men in their 50s and 40–50% in their 70s have prostate cancer but died from other causes. Many men who get tested will thus be found to have high PSA levels. Many will be then biopsied and counselled to have their prostates removed. This will stop them dying from prostate cancer, but the autopsy studies tell us that many of these men would not have died of prostate cancer even if their cancers had never been found. The problem is that there is no reliable way of knowing the benign from the deadly cancers, so overtreatment is rampant.

Second, prostate cancer tends to kill far later in life than other cancers. The average age of death for prostate cancer in Australia is 79.8 years, while the average age for all male cancers combined other than prostate cancer combined is 71.5 – considerably younger. More than half of men who die from the disease are aged 80 or over (average age of death for an Australian man in 2007 was 76 years, so men who die from any cause after that time are already living longer than average); and 82% are aged 70 or more. In 2007, just 2.8% (83 men) who died from the disease were aged less than 60, and 10 (0.1%) were in their 40s.

Men with family histories of prostate cancer are at elevated risk, but it follows that most of these men will have had fathers, uncles and grandfathers who died from the disease very late in life. If these relatives had not died from prostate cancer, many would have died within a few years from other causes because of their advanced age.

So, what's the problem with men wanting to do all they can to avoid dying young, even if the odds are so low (the chance of a man aged 40–44 dying from prostate cancer in a year is a stratospheric one in 250,000 – worse odds than winning the lottery – while for men over 85 it is one in 125)? Thirty years ago, prior to PSA testing being available, our death rate from prostate cancer was 33.4 per 100,000 men. In 2007 it was 31 per 100,000, a decline of 7.2%. The decline probably reflects both early detection and better treatment. Yet over the same period, the incidence of prostate cancer rose 110% from 80.8 per 100,000 to 170 per 100,000, thanks to the aggressive promotion of PSA testing, often by those who stand to benefit financially by its proliferation.

The third major problem is that widespread testing leads to widespread unnecessary surgery and frequent serious complications. Recent data from across NSW show that three years after radical prostatectomy, 77% of men remain impotent and 12% have urinary incontinence compared to 22% and 1% respectively of age-matched men who do not have prostate cancer. Many of these men underwent unnecessary surgery and now live permanently with the consequences. They tend not to talk publicly about these problems. Trite dismissal of the daily lives of thousands of unnecessarily impotent and incontinent men by saying, "You can't have sex in a coffin" is astonishingly arrogant. All this is why earlier this year Richard Ablin who discovered prostate-specific antigen on which the PSA test is based called the promotion of widespread testing "a hugely expensive public health disaster".

In 2009, nine-year results were published from a multi-nation European trial of PSA testing. Dr Peter Bach from New York's Sloan-Kettering Cancer Center summarised the meaning of the trial for a man being treated after testing positive today:

> There is a one in 50 chance that in 2019 or later he will be spared death from a cancer that would otherwise have killed him. And there is a 49 in 50 chance that he will have been treated unnecessarily for a cancer that was never a threat to his life.

Enthusiasts for prostate testing emphasise that the European trial saved lives. It did. But the reduction was from 4.2 to 3.3 deaths per 10,000 person-years.

In 2010, further important results were published from a Swedish trial of prostate cancer screening. These results put a better complexion on the case for screening, finding that as few as 12 men would need to be treated to prevent one prostate cancer death in that population. But expert commentators on that study suggest that Sweden – a nation which has not had comparable proportions to Australia of men tested for prostate cancer – is not an ideal nation from which to draw lessons that would apply here.

Telling someone that they have cancer, particularly when the great majority of men thus diagnosed would have never died from the disease nor had their life in any way affected by the "silent" or indolent cancer inside them, can be deadly serious. We saw that a Swedish study found that the risk of suicide after diagnosis of prostate cancer was 7.4 times higher during the first week after diagnosis and 1.6 times higher during the first year after diagnosis, compared to age-matched men not diagnosed.

Some testing enthusiasts promote the idea that untested men are ignorant or in denial. But many men consciously choose to remain ignorant of their PSA status after reading widely for themselves. Indeed, a Victorian study of GPs aged over 49 found that 55% had not themselves been tested. Celebrities have made wonderful contributions to raising public health awareness, but this carries responsibilities to ensure the public are given the full picture. Promoting prostate cancer testing should emphasise both sides of the issue, to ensure men make fully informed decisions.

We hope that you found the information in this book useful and if so, would encourage you to send it to other men.

The book is available to download as a free PDF file at: hdl.handle.net/2123/6835

References

1. Lee-Jones, C., et al., Fear of cancer recurrence – a literature review and proposed cognitive formulation to explain exacerbation of recurrence fears. *Psychooncology*, 1997, **6**(2): 95–105.

2. Lederer, S.E., Dark victory: cancer and popular Hollywood film. *Bull Hist Med*, 2007, **81**(1): 94–115.

3. Sporn, M.B., The war on cancer: a review. *Ann N Y Acad Sci*, 1997, **833**: 137–46.

4. Reisfield, G.M. and G.R. Wilson, Use of metaphor in the discourse on cancer. *J Clin Oncol*, 2004, **22**(19): 4024–27.

5. Williams Camus, J., Metaphors of cancer in scientific popularization articles in the British press. *Discourse Studies*, 2009, **11**: 465–95.

6. van't Spijker, A., R.W. Trijsburg, and H.J. Duivenvoorden, Psychological sequelae of cancer diagnosis: a meta-analytical review of 58 studies after 1980. *Psychosom Med*, 1997, **59**(3): 280–93.

7. Australian Health Technology Advisory Committee, *Prostate cancer screening*. 1996, Canberra: AGPS.

8. Cancer Council Australia, *National cancer prevention policy 2007–09*. 2007, Sydney: Cancer Council Australia.

9. Royal Australian College of General Practitioners. *Guidelines for preventive activities in general practice 7th edition*. Available from: www.racgp.org.au/redbook/9-7 [Cited 30 Aug 2010].

10. American Cancer Society. *American Cancer Society guidelines for the early detection of cancer*. Available from: www.cancer.org/Healthy/

FindCancerEarly/CancerScreeningGuidelines/american-cancer-society-guidelines-for-the-early-detection-of-cancer?siterea=PED[Cited 30 Aug 2010].

11. BC Cancer Agency. *Prostate cancer*. 2003. Available from: www.bccancer.bc.ca/PPI/Screening/Prostate.htm [Cited 30 Aug 2010].

12. UK National Screening Committee. *The UK NSC policy on prostate cancer screening/PSA testing in men over the age of 50*. Available from: www.screening.nhs.uk/prostatecancer [Cited 30 Aug 2010].

13. US Preventive Services Task Force, Screening for prostate cancer: U.S. Preventive Services Task Force recommendation statement. *Ann Intern Med*, 2008, **149**(3): 185–91.

14. Prostate Cancer Research Foundation of Australia. *PSA/DRE testing for early detection of prostate cancer*. 2006. Available from: www.prostate.org.au/articleLive/attachments/1/PCFA PSA DRE Policy Statement 270706.pdf [Cited 30 Aug 2010].

15. Frankel, S., et al., Screening for prostate cancer. *Lancet Oncol*, 2003, **361**(9363): 1122–28.

16. Holden, C.A., et al., Men in Australia Telephone Survey (MATeS): predictors of men's help-seeking behaviour for reproductive health disorders. *Med J Aust*, 2006, **185**(8): 418–22.

17. Overton P. Secret men's business. *60 Minutes*, 15 Aug 2005. Available from: sixtyminutes.ninemsn.com.au/stories/peteroverton/259324/secret-mens-business [Cited 30 Aug 2010].

18. Schroder, F.H., et al., Screening and prostate-cancer mortality in a randomized European study, [see comment]. *New England Journal of Medicine*, 2009, **360**(13): 1320–28.

19. Margo, J., Cancer test: an expert refusal. *Australian Financial Review*, 6 Feb 2003, pp. 59–60.

20. Commonwealth of Australia, Parliamentary Debates, House of Representatives 5560-15563 (Jim Lloyd) and Editors. 21 June 2003.

21. Anon, The prostate and the apostate (Editorial). *Sydney Morning Herald*, 7 March 2003.

22. Coates, A., Letter. *Sydney Morning Herald*, 10 March 2003.

23. Livingston, P., M. Wakefield, and J.M. Elwood, Community attitudes towards the early detection of cancer in Victoria, Australia. *Aust N Z J Public Health*, 2007, **31**(1): 26–29.

24. Schwartz, L.M., et al., Enthusiasm for cancer screening in the United States. *JAMA*, 2004, **291**(1): 71–78.

25. Gattellari, M. and J.E. Ward, Does evidence-based information about screening for prostate cancer enhance consumer decision-making? A randomised controlled trial. *J Med Screen*, 2003, **10**(1): 27–39.

26. Flood, A.B., et al., The importance of patient preference in the decision to screen for prostate cancer. Prostate Patient Outcomes Research Team. *J Gen Intern Med*, 1996, **11**(6): 342–49.

27. Volk, R.J., A.R. Cass, and S.J. Spann, A randomized controlled trial of shared decision making for prostate cancer screening. *Arch Fam Med*, 1999, **8**(4): 333–40.

28. Wolf, A.M., J.F. Nasser, and J.B. Schorling, The impact of informed consent on patient interest in prostate-specific antigen screening. *Arch Intern Med*, 1996, **156**(12): 1333–36.

29. Davison, B.J., et al., Information and patient participation in screening for prostate cancer. *Patient Educ Couns*, 1999, **37**(3): 255–63.

30. Ferriman, A., Advocates of PSA testing campaign to silence critics. *BMJ*, 2002, **324**(7332): 255.

31. Yamey, G. and M. Wilkes, The PSA storm: questioning cancer screening can be a risky business in America. *BMJ*, 2002, **324**: 431.

32. Movember Australia. *Men's health*. Available from: au.movemberfoundation. com/mens-health/ [Cited 30 Aug 2010].

33. Neal, D.E., PSA testing for prostate cancer improves survival-but can we do better? *Lancet Oncol*, 2010, **11**(8): 702–03.

34. Hugosson, J., et al., Mortality results from the Göteborg randomised population-based prostate-cancer screening trial. *Lancet Oncol*, 2010, **11**(8): 725–32.

35. Waterstreet, C., Movember is for jerks. *Sun Herald*, 21 Nov 2009.

36. Hoffman, R.M., et al., Prostate cancer screening decisions: results from the National Survey of Medical Decisions (DECISIONS Study). *Arch Intern Med*, 2009, **169**(17): 1611–18.

37. Collins, M.M., et al., How common is prostatitis? A national survey of physician visits. *J Urol*, 1998, **159**(4): 1224–28.

38. Krieger, J.N., L. Nyberg, Jr., and J.C. Nickel, NIH consensus definition and classification of prostatitis. *JAMA*, 1999, **282**(3): 236–37.

39. Dimitrakov, J.D., et al., Management of chronic prostatitis/chronic pelvic pain syndrome: an evidence-based approach. *Urology*, 2006, **67**(5): 881–88.

40. Verhamme, K.M., et al., Incidence and prevalence of lower urinary tract symptoms suggestive of benign prostatic hyperplasia in primary care – the Triumph project. *Eur Urol*, 2002, **42**(4): 323–28.

41. Davies, L. and H.G. Welch, Increasing incidence of thyroid cancer in the United States, 1973–2002. *JAMA*, 2006, **295**(18): 2164–67.

42. Breslow, N., et al., Latent carcinoma of prostate at autopsy in seven areas. The International Agency for Research on Cancer, Lyons, France. *Int J Cancer*, 1977, **20**(5): 680–88.

43. Yin, M., et al., Prevalence of incidental prostate cancer in the general population: a study of healthy organ donors. *J Urol*, 2008, **179**(3): 892–95; discussion 895.

44. Australian Institute of Health and Welfare, *Cancer data online*. Available from: www.aihw.gov.au/cancer/data/index.cfm [Cited 30 Aug 2010].

45. Australian Institute of Health and Welfare, *Chronic diseases mortality*. Available from: www.aihw.gov.au/cdarf/data_pages/mortality/index.cfm [Cited 30 Aug 2010].

46. Mackenzie, R., et al., The newsworthiness of cancer in Australian television news. *Med J Aust*, 2008, **189**(3): 155–58.

47. MacKenzie, R., et al., "The news is [not] all good": misrepresentations and inaccuracies in Australian news media reports on prostate cancer screening [see comment]. *Medical Journal of Australia*, 2007, **187**(9): 507–10.

48. MacKenzie, R., et al., 'A matter of faith, not science': analysis of media coverage of prostate cancer screening in Australian news media 2003–2006. *J R Soc Med*, 2007, **100**(11): 513–21.

49. Prostate Cancer Foundation of Australia, *Prostate cancer statistics*. Available from: www.prostate.org.au/articleLive/pages/Prostate-Cancer-Statistics.html [Cited 30 Aug 2010].

50. Australian Institute of Health and Welfare. *Cancer in Australia: an overview, 2008*. Available from: www.aihw.gov.au/publications/can/ca08/ca08.pdf [Cited 30 Aug 2010].

51. AAP, Experts aim to beat prostate cancer fear. *Sydney Morning Herald*, 12 July 2010.

52. Roehl, K.A., et al., Characteristics of patients with familial versus sporadic prostate cancer. *J Urol*, 2006, **176**(6 Pt 1): 2438–42; discussion 2442.

53. Bratt, O., What should a urologist know about hereditary predisposition to prostate cancer? *BJU Int*, 2007, **99**(4): 743–47; discussion 747–48.

54. Wakefield, C.E., et al., Issues faced by unaffected men with a family history of prostate cancer: a multidisciplinary overview. *J Urol*, 2008, **180**(1): 38–46; discussion 46.

55. Zeegers, M., A. Jellema, and H. Ostrer, Empiric risk of prostate carcinoma for relatives of patients with prostate carcinoma. *Cancer*, 2003, **97**(8): 1894–1903.

56. Edwards, S.M. and R.A. Eeles, Unravelling the genetics of prostate cancer. *Am J Med Genet C Semin Med Genet*, 2004, **129C**(1): 65–73.

57. Merrill, R.M. and J.S. Bird, Effect of young age on prostate cancer survival: a population-based assessment (United States). *Cancer Causes Control*, 2002, **13**(5): 435–43.

58. Lin, D.W., M. Porter, and B. Montgomery, Treatment and survival outcomes in young men diagnosed with prostate cancer: a Population-based Cohort Study. *Cancer*, 2009, **115**(13): 2863–71.

59. Key, T.J., et al., The effect of diet on risk of cancer. *Lancet Oncol*, 2002, **360**(9336): 861–68.

60. Cowan, R., et al., The beliefs, and reported and intended behaviors of unaffected men in response to their family history of prostate cancer. *Genet Med*, 2008, **10**(6): 430–38.

61. Muller, D.C., et al., Dietary patterns and prostate cancer risk. *Cancer Epidemiol Biomarkers Prev*, 2009, **18**(11): 3126–29.

62. Boehm, K., et al., Green tea (Camellia sinensis) for the prevention of cancer. *Cochrane Database Syst Rev*, 2009, **3**: CD005004.

63. Etminan, M., B. Takkouche, and F. Caamano-Isorna, The role of tomato products and lycopene in the prevention of prostate cancer: a meta-analysis of observational studies. *Cancer Epidemiol Biomarkers Prev*, 2004, **13**(3): 340–45.

64. Lippman, S.M., et al., Effect of selenium and vitamin E on risk of prostate cancer and other cancers: the Selenium and Vitamin E Cancer Prevention Trial (SELECT). *JAMA*, 2009, **301**(1): 39–51.

65. Thompson, I.M., et al., The influence of finasteride on the development of prostate cancer. *N Engl J Med*, 2003, **349**(3): 215–24.

66. Lucia, M.S., et al., Pathologic characteristics of cancers detected in The Prostate Cancer Prevention Trial: implications for prostate cancer detection and chemoprevention. *Cancer Prev Res (Phila Pa)*, 2008, **1**(3): 167–73.

67. Pinsky, P., H. Parnes, and L. Ford, Estimating rates of true high-grade disease in the prostate cancer prevention trial. *Cancer Prev Res (Phila Pa)*, 2008, **1**(3): 182–86.

68. Leitzmann, M.F., et al., Ejaculation frequency and subsequent risk of prostate cancer. *JAMA*, 2004, **291**(13): 1578–86.

69. Dimitropoulou, P., et al., Sexual activity and prostate cancer risk in men diagnosed at a younger age. *BJU Int*, 2009, **103**(2): 178–85.

70. Lee, I.M., et al., Does physical activity play a role in the prevention of prostate cancer? *Epidemiol Rev*, 2001, **23**(1): 132–37.

71. Harris, R. and L. KN., Screening for Prostate Cancer: An Update of the Evidence for the U.S. Preventive Services Task Force. *Annals of Internal Medicine*, 2002, **137**(11): 915–17.

72. Thompson, I., et al., Prevalence of prostate cancer among men with a prostate-specific antigen level ≤4.0 ng per milliliter. *N Engl J Med*, 2004, **350**(22): 2239–46.

73. Oesterling, J.E., et al., Serum prostate-specific antigen in a community-based population of healthy men. Establishment of age-specific reference ranges. *JAMA*, 1993, **270**(7): 860–64.

74. Albin, R.J., The great prostate mistake. *New York Times*, 9 March 2010.

75. Adapted from: BUPA. Transrectal ultrasound-guided prostate biopsy. 2008. Available from: hcd2.bupa.co.uk/fact_sheets/html/transrectal_prostate_biopsy.html [Cited 30 Aug 2010].

76. Rietbergen, J.B., et al., Complications of transrectal ultrasound-guided systematic sextant biopsies of the prostate: evaluation of complication rates and risk factors within a population-based screening program. *Urology*, 1997, **49**(6): 875–80.

77. Brullet, E., et al., Massive rectal bleeding following transrectal ultrasound-guided prostate biopsy. *Endoscopy*, 2000, **32**(10): 792–95.

78. Borer, A., et al., Fatal Clostridium sordellii ischio-rectal abscess with septicaemia complicating ultrasound-guided transrectal prostate biopsy. *J Infect*, 1999, **38**(2): 128–29.

79. Fall K, et al. Immediate risk for cardiovascular events and suicide following a prostate cancer diagnosis: prospective cohort study. *PLoS Med*, Dec 2009. Available from: www.plosmedicine.org/article/info%3Adoi%2F10.1371%2Fjournal.pmed.1000197 [Cited 30 Aug 2010].

80. Bill-Axelson, A., et al., Suicide risk in men with prostate-specific antigen-detected early prostate cancer: a nationwide population-based cohort study from PCBaSe Sweden. *Eur Urol*, 2010, **57**(3): p. 390–95.

81. Adapted from: US Agency for Healthcare Research and Quality. *Treating cancer: a guide for men with localized prostate cancer*. July 2008. Available

from: www.effectivehealthcare.ahrq.gov/index.cfm/search-for-guides-reviews-and-reports/?pageaction=displayproduct&productID=98 [Cited 30 Aug 2010].

82. Bill-Axelson, A., et al., Radical prostatectomy versus watchful waiting in early prostate cancer. [see comment]. *New England Journal of Medicine*, 2005, **352**(19): 1977–84.

83. Bill-Axelson, A., et al., Radical prostatectomy versus watchful waiting in localized prostate cancer: the Scandinavian prostate cancer group-4 randomized trial. *J Natl Cancer Inst*, 2008, **100**(16): 1144–54.

84. Adapted from: Macmillan Cancer Support. *Radiotherapy for early prostate cancer, 2007.* Available from: www.macmillan.org.uk/Cancerinformation/ Cancertypes/Prostate/Treatmentforearlyprostatecancer/Radiotherapy.aspx [Cited 30 Aug 2010].

85. Adapted from: Roswell Park Cancer Institute. *Prostate cancer.* Available from: www.prostatepros.com/treatment-options/hormonal-therapy-adt-prostate-cancer [Cited 30 Aug 2010].

86. Thompson, I., et al., Guideline for the management of clinically localized prostate cancer: 2007 update. *J Urol*, 2007, **177**(6): 2106–31.

87. Wilt, T.J., et al., Systematic review: comparative effectiveness and harms of treatments for clinically localized prostate cancer. *Ann Intern Med*, 2008, **148**(6): 435–48.

88. Ellison, L.M., J.A. Heaney, and J.D. Birkmeyer, The effect of hospital volume on mortality and resource use after radical prostatectomy. *J Urol*, 2000, **163**(3): 867–69.

89. Yao, S.L. and G. Lu-Yao, Population-based study of relationships between hospital volume of prostatectomies, patient outcomes, and length of hospital stay. *J Natl Cancer Inst*, 1999, **91**(22): 1950–56.

90. Begg, C.B., et al., Variations in morbidity after radical prostatectomy. *N Engl J Med*, 2002, **346**(15): 1138–44.

91. Hunter, K.F., et al., Conservative management for postprostatectomy urinary incontinence. *Cochrane Database Syst Rev*, 2004, **2**: CD001843.

92. Lin, K., et al., Benefits and harms of prostate-specific antigen screening for prostate cancer: an evidence update for the US Preventive Services Task Force. *Ann Intern Med*, 2008, **149**(3): 192–99.

93. Lin K, et al., Benefits and harms of prostate-specific cancer screening: an evidence update for the US Preventive Services Task Force. In *Evidence Synthesis*, No. 63. AHRQ Publication No. 08–05121-EF-1. August 2008, Rockville, Maryland: Agency for Healthcare Research and Quality.

94. Australlian Broadcasting Corporation. *Robots and surgery*. 26 Feb 2009. Available from: www.abc.net.au/rn/futuretense/stories/2009/2500206.htm [Cited 30 Aug 2010].

95. Myprostate.com.au. *Surgery – robotic – da Vinci*. Available from: myprostate.com.au/surgery_da_vinci.htm [Cited 30 Aug 2010].

96. Masters, C., Cutting edge surgery – da Vinci robot's mission is to eliminate cancer. *Daily Telegraph*. 27 May 2006.

97. da Vinci Prostatecomy. Available from: www.davinciprostatectomy.com/index.aspx [Cited 9 Dec 2009].

98. Kooner, R., *Robotic prostate surgery*. St Vincent's Clinic: Sydney.

99. Australian Institute for Robotic Surgery. Available from: www.epworth.org.au/Main-Site/Our-Services/Centres-of-Excellence/Australian-Institute-for-Robotic-Surgery.aspx [Cited 30 Aug 2010].

100. Hu, J., et al., Comparative effectiveness of minimally invasive vs open radical prostatectomy. *JAMA*, 2009, **302**(14): 1557–64.

101. Doumerc, N., et al., Should experienced open prostatic surgeons convert to robotic surgery? The real learning curve for one surgeon over 3 years. *BJU Int*. **106**(3): 378-84.

102. Smith, D.P., et al., Quality of life three years after diagnosis of localised prostate cancer: population based cohort study. *BMJ*, 2009, **339**: b4817.

103. Wilson, G.M.G. and G. Jungner, Principles and practice of screening for disease. *Public Health Papers*, 1968, **34**: 1–163.

104. Keirns, C.C. and S.D. Goold, Patient-centered care and preference-sensitive decision making. *JAMA*, 2009, **302**(16): 1805–06.

105. Andriole, G.L., et al., Mortality results from a randomized prostate-cancer screening trial [see comment]. *New England Journal of Medicine*, 2009, **360**(13): 1310–19.

106. Gøtzsche, P.C. and M. Nielsen, Screening for breast cancer with mammography. *Cochrane Database of Systematic Reviews*, 2009, **4**: CD001877.

107. Kolata G. Prostate test found to save few lives. *New York Times*, 18 Mar 2009. Available from: www.nytimes.com/2009/03/19/health/19cancer.html?_r=2&em&source=cmailer [Cited 30 Aug 2010].

108. Etzioni, R., et al., Overdiagnosis due to prostate-specific antigen screening: lessons from US prostate cancer incidence trends. *J Natl Cancer Inst*, 2002, **94**(13): 981–90.

109. Medd, J.C., et al., Measuring men's opinions of prostate needle biopsy. *ANZ J Surg*, 2005. **75**(8): 662–64.

110. Urological Sociery of Australia and New Zealand. Urological Society of Australia and New Zealand PSA testing policy 2009. Available from: www.usanz.org.au/uploads/29168/ufiles/USANZ_2009_PSA_Testing_Policy_Final1.pdf [Cited 30 Aug 2010].

111. Jorgensen, K.J. and P.C. Gotzsche, Breast screening: fundamental errors in estimate of lives saved by screening. *BMJ*, 2009, **339**: b3359.

112. Morrell, S., et al., Estimates of overdiagnosis of invasive breast cancer associated with screening mammography. *Cancer Causes Control*, 2010, **21**(2): 275–82.

113. Welch, H.G., Overdiagnosis and mammography screening. *BMJ*, 2009, **339**: b1425.

114. Young, J.M. and J.E. Ward, Declining rates of smoking among medical practitioners. *Med J Aust*, 1997, **167**(4): 232.

115. Livingston, P., et al., Knowledge, attitudes and experience associated with testing for prostate cancer: a comparison between male doctors and men in the community. *Intern Med J*, 2002, **32**(5–6): 215–23.

116. Australian Institute of Health and Welfare. *Cancer in Australia*. 2005, 92, Table 46. Available from: www.aihw.gov.au/publications/index.cfm/title/10083 [Cited 30 Aug 2010].

117. Us Too. Prostate Cancer Education and Support. *Corporate supporters*. Available from: www.ustoo.org/Corporate_Sponsors.asp [Cited 9 Dec 2009].

118. Lenzer, J., Lay campaigners for prostate screening are funded by industry. *BMJ*, 2003, **326**(7391): 680.

Index